Caring for Profit

Colleen Fuller is a research associate specializing in public health policy for the Canadian Centre for Policy Alternatives. A long-time researcher and activist around health care issues, she lives in Vancouver.

Caring for Profit

How Corporations Are Taking Over
Canada's Health Care System

Colleen Fuller

NEW STAR BOOKS
VANCOUVER
THE CANADIAN CENTRE FOR POLICY ALTERNATIVES
OTTAWA
1998

New Star Books Ltd.
107 - 3477 Commercial Street
Vancouver, BC
V5N 4E8

Canadian Centre for Policy Alternatives
251 Laurier Avenue West, Ste #804
Ottawa, ON
K1P 5J6

Cover by Working Design
Printed and bound in Canada by Imprimerie Gagné Ltee.,
Louiseville, Québec
1 2 3 4 5   02 01 00 99 98

Publication of the book is made possible by grants from the Canada Council, the British Columbia Arts Council, and the Department of Canadian Heritage Book Publishing Industry Development Program.

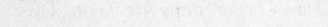

Canadian Cataloguing in Publication Data

Fuller, Colleen, 1952-
    Caring for profit

Copublished by: Canadian Centre for Policy Alternatives
Includes bibliographical references and index.
ISBN 0-921586-59-0

1. Medical care – Canada – Finance.   2. Medical economics – Canada.   3. Health services administration – Canada.   I. Canadian Centre for Policy Alternatives.
II. Title.
RA410.55.C35F84 1998   362.1'0971   C98-910415-X

This book is dedicated to Ben Swankey,

a Canadian leader and comrade in the fight to protect

public pensions and medicare;

and to my parents, Frank and Doris Fuller,

whose unwavering belief in justice and equality

has been instilled in their children,

and in their children's children.

CONTENTS

LIST OF ABBREVIATIONS

AECHC	Alberta Employer Committee on Health Care
AMS	Associated Medical Services
BCMA	British Columbia Medical Association
BCMP	British Columbia Medical Plan
CAC	Consumers' Association of Canada
CANARIE	Canadian Network for the Advancement of Research, Industry and Education
CDMA	Canadian Drug Manufacturers' Association
CHA	Canadian Hospital Associaiton
CHIA	Canadian Health Insurance Association
CHIN	Community Health Information Network
CIBC	Canadian Imperial Bank of Commerce
CIHI	Canadian Institute for Health Information
CLHIA	Canadian Life and Health Insurance Association
CLIOA	Canadian Life Insurance Officers' Association
CMA	Canadian Medical Association
CMDF	Canadian Medical Discoveries Fund
CRO	contract research organizations
DRG	Diagnostic Related Groupings
DSM	disease state management

ECHO   Employer Committee on Health Care-Ontario
EPF   Established Programs Financing Act
FTC   Federal Trade Commission (U.S.)
HIAA   Health Insurance Association of America
HIDS   Hospital Insurance and Diagnostic Services Act
HMO   Health maintenance organization
HRG   Health Resources Group
IBC   Insurance Bureau of Canada
ICBC   Insurance Corporation of British Columbia
IMHC   International Managed Health Care
IT&T   information technology and telecommunications
LHSC   London Health Sciences Centre
MDS   Medical Data Sciences
MDS-HVL   MDS-Hudson Valley Laboratories Inc.
MRC   Medical Research Council
MSAI   Medical Services (Alberta) Incorporated
MSA-BC   Medical Services Association of British Columbia
NHMC   National Healthcare Manufacturing Corp.
OBC   Ontario Blue Cross
OHIP   Ontario Health Insurance Plan
OMA   Ontario Medical Association
OMSIP   Ontario Medical Services Insurance Plan
OTC   over the counter
OWCB   Ontario Workers' Compensation Board
PBM   pharmacy benefits manager
PMAC   Pharmaceutical Manufacturers Association of Canada
PMPRB   Patented Medicine Prices Review Board
ROI   return on investment
SCPS   Saskatchewan College of Physicians and Surgeons
TCMP   Trans-Canada Medical Plan
TML   Toronto Medical Laboratories
TTH   The Toronto Hospital
WBGH   Washington (D.C.) Business Group on Health
WCB   Workers' Compensation Board

FOREWORD

In 1996, we decided to commission research on the role of the for-profit health industry in Canada's health care system. We were concerned that government funding cutbacks in a climate of deregulation and privatization suggested a likely corporate takeover, and that the changes underway were weakening the foundations of public health care. Moreover, we were concerned that there was hardly any coverage of the issue in the mainstream media, and consequently little public awareness of what was happening.

Our appeal for funding to undertake this research project, assisted by a formal endorsement from the Canadian Health Coalition, drew a positive response from across the country. The following organizations provided financial assistance: the Alberta Teacher's Association, the British Columbia Nurses' Union, the Canadian Union of Public Employees, the Communications, Energy and Paper Workers Union, the Hospital Employees Union of British Columbia, the National Federation of Nurses' Unions, the National Union of Public and General Employees, the Public Service Alliance of Canada, the Service Employees International Union, the Saskatchewan Union of Nurses, and the United Steelworkers of America. In casting about for the right person to do this work, we learned that Colleen Fuller, one of the country's leading health policy analysts, was interested and available. To our delight she agreed to take on the challenge.

The completion of this project has taken much longer than we originally anticipated, but it has been worth the wait. *Caring for Profit* is a brilliant exposé of the corporate players (and their allies in government) behind the push to transform our health system into a U.S.-style system dominated by "free market" competition.

Caring for Profit documents how we as a society fought for and achieved a universal, not-for-profit, publicly-financed health care system. It reveals, with a depth and clarity not previously available to the Canadian public, the corporate forces now subverting the system, their strategies and the enormous financial stakes; and it shows us what we have to do to change direction.

Canadians have been kept in the dark about how and why our health care system is under threat. This book takes a giant "kick at the darkness," providing the means for Canadians to take action to reclaim and improve their health care system.

Bruce Campbell
Executive Director,
Canadian Centre for Policy Alternatives
Ottawa, October 1998

PREFACE

When I began this book I thought privatization in Canada's health sector was a straightforward issue, something I could present in short order. But privatization is much more complicated than I had imagined, with many faces and manifestations, many champions and many detractors. It is a difficult subject for Canadians to learn about, not least because information about what politicians and corporations are doing to health care is harder and harder to come by. Yet information is essential if Canadians are to have any control over what happens to our health-care system. We need to judge truth from fiction – and in health care there is a lot of fiction.

Increasingly, Canadians are left in the dark about the objectives of and the rationale behind policy changes, not to mention the policy changes themselves. But the changes occurring on the public policy front are not the only things we need to know about. We also need to know about health corporations: their sources of revenue and profits, their directors, major investors, global and political links, and their track records in other countries, particularly in the United States.

Information and analysis are vital; however, they mean little if we ignore what we feel and know is being experienced by ourselves, our families, and our communities. Sometimes we just have to pause and listen to our own true voices. If we feel that health-care in our communities could be better, we have to trust those perceptions and use them as the springboard into the future.

Many unions and organizations contributed to *Caring for Profit*. In particular I would like to thank the Canadian Centre for Policy Alternatives, which believed that a book on health-care privatization would be useful (and believed that I could write it), and both the members and staff of the Canadian Union of Public Employees, the Hospital Employees' Union, the Nova Scotia Government Employees' Union, and the Service Employees International Union, all of whom were vital to this project. The Canadian Health Coalition and its provincial counterparts contributed ideas and information that, I hope, are reflected in this book. I owe a great debt, as well, to Bruce Campbell of the CCPA who originally approached me about this project, and who supported me every step along what turned out to be a long road; and to my good friend Rolf Maurer of New Star Books.

So many people helped me in so many different ways, I hardly know where to begin in expressing my thanks. Audrey McClellan brought her phenomenal editorial skills and her indefatigable and querying mind to this project. Pat and Hugh Armstrong, Seth Klein, Ben Swankey, Govind Sundram, Nick DiCarlo, Irene Jansen, Mike Old, Mike McBane, Wendy Armstrong, Margi Blamey, and Marcy Cohen were among those who read early versions of the manuscript, in whole or in part, and who provided me with such good advice, helped me fill out the picture of health, and encouraged me to keep going. Kathy McLennan, Cynthia Williams, Sandra Sorensen, Ian Johnson, Margot Young, Laura Sky, Laurel Ritchie, Yukie Kurahashi, Stan Marshall, Neil Monckton and Adrianna Tetley were among those who offered insights, information, and suggestions and who supported me personally and professionally while I punched endlessly away on the computer.

And finally I thank John Calvert for reaching into what seems an endless well of patience and love, and for sharing that with me even when I was mean and wicked.

Colleen Fuller
Victoria, B.C., October 1998

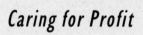

Caring for Profit

Introduction

More than thirty years after Canadians achieved universal, nonprofit, publicly administered health insurance, we have reached a crossroads. Down one branch of the divided road lies a publicly funded health system most of us regard as a cornerstone of our culture and history, one in which we and our children find the support we need to stay healthy, the high-quality care we need when we are ill, and the means to maintain such a system fairly and equitably. Down the alternate route is a profit-oriented, urban, health industry that is not locally based but is integrated across national boundaries and dominated by a handful of global corporations, an industry in which most of us participate at great cost, retaining the freedom to choose between bankruptcy and poor health. Neither option looks like the Canadian health-care system of the 1990s.

Let's take a moment to walk through the system of today. A Canadian patient – I'll call her Doris – enters the world of health care by way of the doctor's office. Since most physicians in Canada are private entrepreneurs, this first point of contact is in the private sector, although her doctor's fees are paid by a public health plan. Her journey through the system will resemble a patchwork quilt of for-profit and not-for-profit, public and private health-service providers. If she requires a blood test, Doris's family doctor likely will refer her to a private, for-profit laboratory, possibly one in which he himself is an investor. The lab fees, like the doctor's, will be paid by the public plan.

If her doctor concludes she needs surgery, Doris may be placed on a waiting list until the surgeon is available. It may be a long wait because the surgeon has a preference for patients covered by private insurance, which pays him higher fees than the public plan, so Doris gets bumped to the back of the line. Once she is admitted to hospital for the surgery, all of the services she requires are provided by the nonprofit, publicly funded but privately administered hospital and are paid for by the public health plan.

The government of the province where Doris lives has been trying to reduce public health expenditures, so Doris's hospital has had its budget cut and has been downsizing. There are fewer staff, and patients are being released sooner so the hospital can save money. When she is released, Doris needs a physiotherapist, but the hospital has closed its outpatient rehabilitation department. Therefore, her doctor refers her to a for-profit rehab company that is able to provide the service. If Doris is on an extended health plan provided by her employer, the private physiotherapy services will be wholly or partially paid for by a private insurance company. If she's not on extended benefits, in some parts of Canada the cost of physiotherapy will be shared between Doris and her public health plan, while in other parts of the country Doris will pay the whole shot herself. Luckily, she lives in a province that covers physio services, even though the physiotherapist is allowed to charge a $10 user fee for each visit. Doris can manage that.

Since Doris was not fully recovered from her operation when she was discharged from the hospital, she needs support when she gets home in addition to the physiotherapy sessions. Unless home care or nursing services are included in her extended health plan, she will have to pay whatever charges are billed to her by the private company she has been referred to by her doctor, hospital, insurer, or other adviser. Doris is not disabled or over sixty-five years old, so she also will have to pay for the drugs her doctor has prescribed, either the full price or a partial amount depending on whether she is privately insured, whether the drug is included on her plan, and whether her insurer approves of the prescription. Because she was not injured on the job, if Doris's illness continues for a lengthy period and she is unable to return to work, she will be ineligible for wage replacement from the Workers' Compensation Board and is likely to suffer a loss of income.

Doris is a champion of medicare, but her provincial government is not as enthusiastic as it used to be. Health costs have been rising faster than the cost of living and the province is removing, or "delisting," services (for example, the outpatient physiotherapy services) from the public health plan. In spite of these cuts, Doris knows that most of the fare for her journey through the health-care system was paid for by the provincial government, that some of it was paid for by her extended health plan, and that the balance (for home care and deductibles for her drugs) came out of her own pocket. But Doris doesn't know that a large number of shareholders and investors – a number that is growing rapidly in Canada – all made the journey with her, and each one took a few dollars – or a few thousand dollars – out of the fare for themselves. The doctor, the lab, the physiotherapy company, the private nurse – in fact, all of the providers, with the exception of the nonprofit society that runs the hospital – increased their profit margins when Doris became ill.

How did we get to this crossroads? Why is public health insurance – what William Lyon Mackenzie King referred to in 1918 as "a means ... to bring about a wider measure of social justice" – in crisis and health care a battlefield between those who support profit making as a sacred right and those who defend medicare as a sacred trust?

Medicare's history is full of heroism and pettiness, generosity and greed, alliances and individual actions. In this respect, little has changed. But today the stakes in the ongoing tug-of-war between a public, nonprofit health-care system and a private, for-profit one are higher than they've ever been. Canadians spent more than $76.6 billion on health care in 1997, approximately 68 percent of that through their governments and the remainder through individual purchases of drugs, medical equipment, home care, insurance, and other products and services. Overall health expenditures increased by 1.4 percent from 1995 to 1997, a minuscule rise compared to an average increase of 11.2 percent annually from 1975 to 1991. However, the most dramatic change has occurred in the split between public and private per capita spending in Canada. In 1991 Canadians spent an average of $606 each in the private health sector and paid $1761 each in taxes that were used for publicly insured or provided services such as hospital and physician care. By 1997 Canadians spent $790 each in the private sector, an increase of 30 percent, while public-sector expenditures averaged $1737 each, a decrease of 1.6 percent. The increase in the amount of money Canadians spent on health services coincided with a decrease in individuals' real spending power.[1]

The sharp rise in private health expenditures is taking place during a period characterized by low rates of inflation, increased privatization, federal and provincial health funding cuts, deregulation, and limits placed on public health plans. The figures raise many questions about what governments and public policy makers are doing to health care and about who exactly they are doing it for. There is no doubt that Canada's private health industry has been the main beneficiary of federal and provincial health strategies during the past decade. While 68 percent of the overall $76.6 billion health tab is paid by all levels of government, a greater portion of it is going to purchase drugs and services from large and small corporations, while the availability of services in the nonprofit sector is declining. Drugs and doctors, both in the private sector, together consume 30 percent of the public health dollar.

World expenditures for health-care services – excluding medical supplies, biotechnology, and information technology – are more than US$3 trillion annually, but these resources are not distributed equitably either among nations or within nations. Canada's portion of world health expenditures is 2.5 percent, compared to more than 30 percent consumed by Americans, more than 12 percent by all of Asia, and 25 percent by all the countries of Europe. The remaining one third is divided unevenly among the rest of the world's population. More than half of the world's health-care money is spent by governments to provide services directly or indirectly, with the remaining amount spent by individuals or employers for services provided by the private sector. That latter portion is expected to increase as governments, under pressure from the International Monetary Fund (IMF), the World Bank, and trade agendas such as the North American Free Trade Agreement (NAFTA), privatize health or insurance services, creating a more hospitable climate for investors.

In the last decade, the pattern of problems and changes in Canada's health-care sector has been remarkably similar to that in dozens of countries around the globe. Patients in both industrialized and developing countries face longer and longer waits for overburdened public services, and turn to a burgeoning private sector if they can afford it. Governments have cut or eliminated public funding of hospital care, forcing patients to depend on already stretched family members, especially women. Authority and funding have devolved from national to regional to local levels, fragmenting public control, while private health care is concentrating in fewer and more distant hands. Hospitals from Halifax to Manila have been reengineered to deliver standardized health-care regimes that work on young, healthy, white males in Chicago or San Francisco. For-profit companies have taken over small and medium-sized nonprofit entities, both public and private, and are now offering for-profit health care in countries around the world.

Is there a link between domestic policies that promote privatization and the globalization of large, mainly American and European, health-care corporations? Absolutely. Privatization is a public policy goal of many governments around the globe, one that is frequently at the top of the agenda during high-level trade talks, international summits, and economic forums where strategies, contacts, and anecdotes are exchanged. When international trade deals are signed they promise, among other things, to further the domestic opportunities for global corporations. It is taken for granted that corporate lobbyists and advisers will be on hand to assist politicians and bureaucrats in their deliberations. The worldwide trend to deregulate economies, privatize public services, and pave the way for wealthy investors who want to become wealthier is not a mere stroke of luck. But neither is it a conspiracy. It is, rather, a goal with a plan.

Health care that would serve the needs of Canadians is being replaced by those services that will enhance the profits of corporate investors in the health industry. This direction is supported – and increasingly required – by Canada's major trading partner, the United States, and by a growing number of trade agreements signed by Ottawa that limit Canadians' rights and powers over their health care and their health. It is hard to credit the argument that there is no grand design being pursued by the global corporations whose names and logos are coming to dominate the health industries around the world. There simply is too much evidence to the contrary.

It can hardly be a coincidence, for example, that the removal of foreign ownership restrictions in the Filipino insurance market beginning in 1995 was a mirror-image of the steps taken by Canada five years earlier to meet the new rules of free trade, signalling the start of insurance company mergers, acquisitions, and Confederation Lifestyle collapses. Nor is it plausible that the introduction of twenty-year patents to protect giant pharmaceutical manufacturers from generic competitors in Canada – a move that increased Canada's drug costs from the lowest to the second highest in the industrial world – is unrelated to the decisions of governments in India and other countries to do likewise. Hospitals in both Nicaragua and Canada are closing in favour of "community-based alternatives," many of which are being acquired by foreign multinationals that provide poorer standards of care and underpay their caregivers. It is not happenstance but is plotted out in structural adjustment programs, trade deals, and, if necessary, constitutional amendments.

If corporations don't actually conspire to cash in on health care, they do carry out careful planning to further their common ends, and these ends are not shared by the Canadian people. There are joint efforts by investors and their allies in provincial and federal governments (some of whom are future directors of the same companies benefitting from privatization) to dismantle a great public enterprise and create a profitable private health industry – and to manage public opinion so that the anger of Canadians does not erupt like a volcano.

It may not be a conspiracy, but the takeover of public and nonprofit health-care services, the acquisition of small and medium-sized Canadian companies by large corporations, and the refusal or inability of federal and provincial governments to intervene on behalf of citizens bear a chilling resemblance to the demise of another great public endeavour – the highly efficient, nonpolluting, affordable, electric streetcar system that ran in the United States during the early years of this century. A look back at the systematic replacement of streetcars with private automobiles is instructive for those concerned about health care.

Beginning in the 1920s, General Motors president Alfred Sloan and top company executives masterminded a scheme to create a consumer market for automobiles in the United States. At the time, nine out of ten people relied on the trolley networks that crisscrossed cities across the country. GM first purchased and then dismantled the nation's trolley companies, ripping up tracks and setting bonfires composed of rail cars. In thirty short years GM succeeded in destroying a mass-transit infrastructure that would cost many billions of dollars to resurrect – more money than municipal governments could raise. The trolley cars were replaced with GM's diesel-fuelled buses, service was cut back, air pollution increased, and people began buying cars. National Car Lines (NCL), a company controlled and funded by GM, soon operated public transit in eighty cities. A propaganda campaign – including the slogan "What's good for General Motors is good for America" – was mounted, depicting private automobiles as a modern, timesaving alternative to supposedly inefficient, slow, public transportation systems defended by behind-the-times municipal authorities and citizens.

In the 1950s the powerful American highway lobby launched an aggressive campaign for public funds to underwrite the construction of an interstate road system. Charles Wilson, GM's president at that time, was appointed Secretary of Defense in 1953, and he argued that a national highway system was a national security issue. Federal Highway Administrator Francis DuPont, a member of GM's largest shareholder family, was given a green light and $50 billion to begin construction on the interstate highway system. Across the United States, people fought plans to build freeways through their towns and cities, but Washington's ear was attuned only to the corporate sector.

In the 1960s, GM, NCL, Standard Oil, and Firestone were convicted in an anti-trust suit of conspiring to destroy public transportation in the United States. GM was fined $5000, far short of the hundreds of billions needed by pollution-choked cities to rebuild an electric trolley system and reduce reliance on private cars as the main mode of transportation. The deed was done, the wrong branch had been chosen at the crossroad, and it had become too costly to turn back.[2]

Wealthy investors and corporate executives are long-term thinkers, and much of their thinking focusses on maintaining or, if necessary, creating an environment in which corporate entities can successfully fulfill the task they were established to achieve. The mandate of all corporations is to earn profits, and the job of a corporate executive is to organize only those activities that will return profits to the people who invest in his or her company. Canada's emerging health industry is the product of such long-term plans, of strategic alliances developed in boardrooms, at conferences, and over cocktails, and of relationships forged among the members of corporate elites who often rub elbows on more than one board and in more than one industry. These connections are both formal and informal – based on contractual undertakings or joint ventures, shared ideologies or complementary interests.

Health company investors and executives are careful to portray themselves and the corporations they represent as enthusiastic champions of high-quality, affordable care and universal accessibility. Although they often assign moral characteristics to their companies, such entities are in fact amoral. A "good" corporation is simply one that earns a high rate of return, just as a "good" table is one that stands firmly on its four legs. Similarly, a company that registers low profit margins because it upholds the values of the community is "bad," just as a table that can't stay up is worthless. Health corporation executives who care more for patients than for profits are neglecting their mandate; they are shirking their responsibility to investors, and such conduct is subject to the scrutiny and the discipline of the market.

Morality, however, is a key to understanding how and why the Canadian people chose to remove financial and other barriers to the health-care system. The corporate imperative to return high profits to investors was identified by an overwhelming majority of the nation's people as a moral question during the long years leading up to the introduction of medicare. Simply put, Canadians viewed the idea of making money from the misfortunes of the sick or the needs of the disabled – whether themselves or their neighbours – with repugnance. Thus the struggle that led to the establishment of medicare was fought on the grounds of compassion, equity, access, and fairness, where it remains to this day.

A crossroads is a difficult place to be. We can't stand still and we can't take two different routes at the same time. One direction promises to lead us towards a market-driven system of health care. The other will build on the achievements of our predecessors. To move ahead with confidence, Canadians must learn more about where we've come from and where we are today.

The choices are difficult, but the times are interesting, and Canadians, as ever, are stubborn about health care. As much as anything else, this will be a deciding factor in the years ahead.

ONE

Historical Alliances

The creation of Canada's medicare system was the result of a long struggle, countless compromises, and a rejection by many millions of people of what existed at the time, in favour of what could be. The move towards equitable access to hospital and physician services came late to Canada in comparison to most countries in Europe and the United Kingdom, where some form of public health delivery or insurance was being established by the 1920s. And it was not an easy transition from a system in which health was viewed as a private affair to one that entrusted government with the responsibility for ensuring that all Canadians, regardless of how much money or what kind of illness they had, obtained access to medical care.

The debate on what role, if any, government should assume in ensuring the health of its citizens began in earnest during World War I, when the issue was pushed onto the national agenda by groups fighting for social benefits ranging from sewage treatment facilities to public education. Health care was denied to many millions of Canadian families because they could not afford to pay the price, but even those who had money experienced problems because there were few trained doctors and even fewer adequately staffed and sanitary hospitals. As provincial legislatures grappled with the complexities surrounding public and private provision of health services, Canadians initiated a national debate about a national health program. Organizations representing workers, farmers, women, large and small businesses, doctors, and hospitals began mobilizing on one side of the question or the other. What is striking about these early debates is the way groups and individuals positioned themselves around the issue of a national health program and how similar their positions are today.

While a broad segment of Canadian society supported a public health program, there were deep divisions about whether such a scheme should be universal or for low-income earners only, about whether doctors should be paid on a fee-for-service or salaried basis, and about the appropriate role of the state in insuring or providing health care services. These divisions ran like a fault line that separated, on one side, organized medicine, big business, and private insurers – most of whom were determined to design and expand a medical system in which they could provide a minimum of care at a maximum rate of return – and on the other side, the overwhelming majority of Canadians who embraced the principles of universal access to and nonprofit delivery of services from the start.

The birth of medicare was constrained and influenced by a number of factors unique to Canada. The constitutional arrangements in Canada's federated system seemed to conflict with the idea of and the demand for a national health care program. To this day there are no constitutional answers to the question "Which level of government has jurisdiction over health and health care?" The British North America Act, Canada's constitution at the time, did not allocate explicit legislative authority over health care to any level of government, noting only that Ottawa was responsible for "quarantine and the establishment and maintenance of marine hospitals," while provinces were to establish, maintain, and manage "hospitals, asylums, charities and eleemosynary [charitable] institutions."

In 1940 the Rowell-Sirois Royal Commission on Dominion-Provincial Relations, struck to examine constitutional responsibilities in Canada, recognized the ambiguity of the BNA Act on the question of health care. The commissioners attempted to clarify the matter, recommending that the provinces should accept responsibility for designing "the method of providing state medical services" to low-income and indigent Canadians, whether the method chosen was health insurance or direct provision of such services, a distinction that was not elaborated upon. The commission's report also recommended that the provinces be given responsibility for health insurance, although they qualified this somewhat by adding, "It is not improbable that, in the course of time ... conditions would warrant national Health Insurance or a national system of Workmen's Compensation. It would, therefore, seem desirable that rigidity in the matter of jurisdiction should be avoided."

The often bitter disputes between Ottawa and the provinces about funding and the provision of health services can be traced to these early actors who were unable to resolve the question of jurisdiction. These tensions often have been used by the opponents of medicare to manipulate provincial fears of federal meddling and heavy-handedness in health care – an area that depends on a high degree of cooperation between the two levels of government.

But if the constitutional question of who will fund health care and under what criteria causes problems, so too does the question of what method of funding will be used. After World War II, when these issues were being examined in detail, Canadians looked at two clear alternatives: publicly or privately funded health care. They opted for a public model. The method of funding Canadians' access to health care received far less attention, even though it was an issue of equal importance. Here, too, there were two alternatives: the first was public health insurance to fund the private provision of services; the second, referred to pejoratively as "state medicine," was a public health system paid for and run by the state, similar to Canada's public education system. All of these were hard choices confronting the public.

Among industrialized countries (with the exception of the U.S.), health-care systems fall into two broad categories according to the financing structure used to support them. The first is known as the Beveridge model, a tax-based system named after Lord Beveridge, creator of the National Health Service in Britain. The second, called the Bismarck model, is associated with the German system of social insurance and is used in most German-speaking countries as well as in France and the Netherlands. These different financing arrangements influence how health services are organized, and they were carefully studied by policymakers in Canada as the country moved towards implementing medicare in the 1960s.

In Germany, since the 1920s, the working population has been covered by mandatory private health insurance, with the unemployed covered by public programs. Insurers receive a payroll tax paid by workers and employers on a 50-50 split and amounting to between 8 and 16 percent of wages. Patients can choose their own doctors, who are paid on a fee-for-service basis. Doctors are private entrepreneurs and negotiate their fees with the insurance companies that represent the doctors' patients. Hospitals are private and nonprofit, but many nonacute-care services are provided in a competitive, highly regulated, for-profit marketplace.

Tax-based systems, as the name implies, are funded by tax revenues and place a greater emphasis on primary care, prevention, home care, and sheltered housing. Doctors are paid on a salaried or capitated (i.e., a set amount per patient) basis. Most services, both hospital and non-hospital, are located in the public sector and are more coordinated than competitive. Health insurance is not required to access services, and services are not paid for on an insured, item-by-item basis. Typically, tax-based models are highly integrated; because both payer and provider are one and the same, services can be organized and managed in a more continuous and coherent manner.

Canada developed a hybrid system known as "medicare" (in the United States it is referred to as the "single payer" system). It is a tax-based public insurance system that pays for health services supplied mainly by the private sector. Over 95 percent of hospitals in Canada operate as private, nonprofit entities run by community boards, voluntary organizations, or municipalities. Hospitals are funded by governments to provide publicly insured hospital care, which often does not include the full spectrum of outpatient rehab, counselling, nursing, home care, and dental or other health services. Most doctors are private entrepreneurs who, through their professional organizations, negotiate fee-for-service payment levels with provincial governments.

The delivery of primary and preventive care is disorganized, under-funded, and, like outpatient services generally, threatened by a grow-ing for-profit health industry.

The public insurance system is augmented by private plans that receive premiums from individuals and employers, and by a system of workers' compensation that pays for health services for workers injured or disabled on the job.

Most countries that have a tax-based health system devote two to three percentage points less of Gross Domestic Product (GDP) to health costs than do countries with social insurance schemes. There is one notable exception to this statistic: Canada. In most tax-based systems the public both pays for and provides the services, producing cost-savings and efficiencies. Canada's model of public payment and pri-vate provision (called a payer-provider split) originally let Canadians build on the principles of nonprofit delivery to establish an equitable health system. But as the role of for-profit businesses has expanded, the split between payer and provider has burdened Canadians with unnecessarily high costs. Not only is Canada's system more costly than it needs to be, but it also is fragmented at the funding allocation, the delivery, and the policy levels.

Canada's health financing arrangements do not allow the govern-ments that fund the system to manage services provided by private entities or to prevent private companies from duplicating services delivered in the hospital sector. Governments cannot tell companies to locate in sparsely populated rural communities or to ensure that a full spectrum of population health needs are met, because the mandate of private corporations is to provide a service if the service provides a healthy return on investment — no more and no less. Canada's system of insured services also allows governments to pay only for services that are "medically necessary," a pseudo-scientific term that is increasingly used to camouflage the political considerations behind the removal or delisting of medical procedures from provincial health plans.

Canada's public health insurance model has failed to achieve the full benefits one would normally expect to see in a tax-supported health system. These include the benefits of continuity, integration, salaried physicians, and lower GDP expenditures, all of which could be gained without the painful cuts in funding and services that we are seeing today. These benefits could be realized if Canadians integrated private providers with public payers, that is, if the provision or delivery of health care was moved out of the private sector.

Instead we are moving in the opposite direction. Public control over where the health dollar goes (and for what) is regionalized and fragmented, while the private sector is consolidating and integrating into powerful national and global entities.

To see how we got to this point, it's necessary to go back to the beginning, to the first stirrings of the concept of public health insurance in Canada, and watch the development of the present system and the alliances formed to aid or obstruct it.

The beginnings of Canadian health insurance

The decision to establish a public health insurance system reflected the experiences of Canadians over nearly three centuries, beginning in 1665 in Montreal, when a contract was drawn between the city's master surgeon and a group of families for the provision of medical services. Seven years later, North America's first in-hospital services contract was signed between the Mother Superior of Montreal's Dames Religieuses Hospitalieres and two master surgeons who promised to "well and truly serve the hospital of Ville-Marie, to treat, dress and physic all the sick persons who may be there ... for periods of three months each in turn and to visit such sick persons assiduously at about seven o'clock each morning and at such other hours as may be necessary ... "

But it was Nova Scotia's Provincial Workers' Association, representing miners in the Glace Bay colliery, that won the first formal agreement with an employer in 1883 for a "medical check-off" system that allowed workers to use physician and hospital services of their choosing. (Interestingly, the doctors received a set fee for each patient – a system called capitation – rather than for each service.) The wage deductions – probably the first time check-off of any kind was instituted in Canada – were compulsory for all employees of the mining company, even though the practice was not legally sanctioned until

1903. This method was later adopted in other mining and logging communities across the country, notably in Timmins, Ontario, and in Trail, Nanaimo, Chemainus, and Port Alberni, British Columbia.

In 1878 St. Joseph's Hospital in Victoria, B.C., became the first hospital in Canada to offer a prepaid health plan for "gratuitous admission, visits of the doctor at reduced rates and medicines free of charge ... for a monthly subscription fee of one dollar." Eleven years later the Medicine Hat General Hospital in what was then the Northwest Territories sponsored an insurance scheme to assist in its efforts to secure operating revenues. Residents could buy a hospital insurance ticket for five dollars a year entitling them to "lodge, board and ... nurse and medical attendance." This idea eventually spread to the Maritimes, where the Hôtel Dieu in Chatham, New Brunswick, introduced "admission tickets" in 1907 when the hospitalization of loggers "who had either been injured in the woods or there contracted some malady" increased.

These early efforts protected workers from some of the consequences of job-related injuries and illness and gave rise in the new century to two separate but related (and often overlapping) demands by unions organizing across Canada. Trade unions wanted a system of workers' compensation with wage replacement during convalescence, as well as health benefits covering physician services and hospitalization for workers and their dependants regardless of where an illness originated. These demands for "sickness insurance" were based, in large part, on the experiences of Canada's emerging industrial working class, which confronted dangerous and often lethal conditions of work, particularly in the logging, railway, and mining industries.

The struggle during the last century for safe working conditions met with ferocious opposition from employers, who resisted workers' demands (and provincial regulations where they existed) despite the annual death toll. Canada's entry into World War I brought about increased pressure for safe workplaces and a system of workers' compensation that would adequately protect the casualties on the frontlines of production. These efforts were coupled with demands for a public scheme to cover the costs of health care associated with sickness – whether work related or not. As we shall see, decades would pass before governments finally acted.

On the Prairies, poverty and low farm incomes led families to experiment with prepaid hospital services before the turn of the century. By 1914 several medical and hospital programs had emerged in Alberta, Saskatchewan, and Manitoba. The first was the municipal hospital care system for indigents, financed by general tax revenues. A number of towns began paying hospital fees for all residents, supported by property taxes.

Prairie residents also had to deal with the question of how to attract and keep doctors in rural areas where support services were limited, as were opportunities to earn a reasonable income. This gave rise to the municipal doctor system in the three provinces, which offered rural physicians an annual salary in exchange for medical services. By the mid-1930s, seventy-five Prairie municipalities operated the program, most of them in Saskatchewan.

The third program was known as the union hospital system. Towns, villages, and rural municipalities combined in districts to build, administer, and manage "Union Hospitals" during World War I. These hospitals negotiated with municipal governments for a fixed annual contribution so they could provide services to "indigents" in the district.

Although there were many thousands of people involved in provincial and national debates about health insurance, those who were organized had the most impact. Workers, farmers, social activists, physicians, insurers, and investors were joining together to secure or to defeat medicare. Alliances, some of which endure to this day, were formed on one side of the question or the other to press their case before the public and provincial and federal governments. Farmers, workers, and the poor all had compelling reasons to support government-sponsored health care and often had direct and positive experiences with a more cooperative approach. But they confronted an equally determined opposition committed to a free enterprise, profit-based model. Medicare's opponents numbered fewer than its supporters, but they included some of the most powerful organizations in the country – chambers of commerce and boards of trade, manufacturers, industrialists, and organized physicians, among others.

The stock market crash of October 1929 and the ensuing economic crisis temporarily overshadowed provincial and national debates on health care. Under Canadian law, responsibility for the mounting numbers of poor people, and that included the sick poor, fell to municipalities, many of which were on the verge of, or were actually declaring, bankruptcy. While relief was grudgingly provided to "indigents" for food, clothing, and shelter, health care, like unemployment insurance, usually was not. In every municipality the growing lines of poor people at soup kitchens and relief agencies were complemented by the growing queues of sick women, men, and children applying to civic authorities for admittance to municipal hospitals where they would be cared for free of charge if they faced a medical emergency. If they were turned away there, they were forced to seek private charity for outpatient or physician services. If that appeal failed, they were left to run from one strange doctor to another, leaving a trail of unpaid medical bills behind them.

The precipitous drop in the income of Canadians during the Depression was felt in the country's medical community as well. During the 1920s, physician incomes ranged from a low of $5000 a year for general practitioners in rural communities to over $11,000 a year for urban specialists. This compared favourably with an average annual income for industrial workers in Canada barely above $1000. During the Hungry Thirties, however, physicians saw their revenues sharply decrease because their patients often went without medical services, an unaffordable luxury item in the family budget.

Doctors found themselves doing more charity work for the poor, for which they received no payment, as well as seeing a growing number of patients unable to pay for non-charity work already rendered. Many doctors who abhorred the conditions imposed by tight-fisted governments during the Depression joined in campaigns led by groups and individuals such as Dr. Norman Bethune and his colleagues in Montreal. In cities across Canada they called for medical relief or public health insurance for the poor. In Winnipeg, doctors launched a strike that lasted for seven months in 1933, ending only when the city council agreed to set up a medical relief plan. In Ontario, the provincial government announced in 1932 that it would assist any municipality with a medical relief scheme that would meet some of the doctors' demands, but it excluded in-hospital care from the amount of the subsidy. Many doctors combined their heartfelt compassion for the poor with their own desire for a source of needed revenue in similar campaigns, some of which were successful. Physician incomes had fallen by as much as 72 percent in Saskatchewan and more than 40 percent in British Columbia.

Low physician incomes led the Canadian Medical Association (CMA) to launch an important internal debate about its position on a national health insurance scheme. This was one of many debates the CMA, along with its provincial divisions, conducted over a period of more than thirty years, from 1917 to 1949, during which it alternately expressed great enthusiasm for state-sponsored health insurance and loathing for socialized medicine. But regardless of whether the CMA accepted a public health insurance model "in principle," in practice the organization actively and vehemently opposed each attempt by both federal and provincial governments to introduce such a system. By the time Saskatchewan moved to introduce North America's first medicare scheme in the 1950s, the CMA had finally and firmly abandoned its ambiguity and come out in favour of privately financed, privately provided health care with, if necessary, a separate tier funded by government for the poor.

Public health insurance in British Columbia, 1936

The first attempt to introduce a health insurance scheme in Canada occurred in British Columbia in 1936. A Royal Commission had proposed a provincial plan that would cover all medical services, hospitalization, drugs and appliances, and, eventually, dental care. There was general support for the idea – with the exception of the Vancouver *Sun*, which opposed health insurance as "unsound morally and socially," and wealthy businessmen who opposed any progressive social reform that might increase the deficit.

When the new Liberal government introduced legislation establishing public health insurance in March 1936, many of the key elements in the Commission's report were missing, including coverage for the unemployed poor (although low-wage earners would still be eligible).

The Liberals were feeling pressure from many sides. A new political party, the Cooperative Commonwealth Federation (CCF), with strong backing from the province's working-class voters, now sat on the Opposition benches of the B.C. legislature. The CCF demanded a universal health insurance plan for all British Columbians that would be funded from general revenues rather than through premiums and payroll deductions. This position was in general accord with the demands of a majority of British Columbians including low-wage workers, unions, women's groups, churches, and farmers. Though the CCF lent its support to the government's scaled-back version, it viewed the plan as only a first step towards a public health system.

The CMA had responded warmly to the report of the Royal Commission that led to B.C.'s legislative initiative. In 1934 it released a detailed policy statement that embraced public health insurance in principle; shortly after that the organization gave its initial approval to the commission's report. As well, the CMA had been consulted extensively when the legislation was being written, and its proposals were almost completely incorporated into the draft presented to the legislature in March 1935. But when the Liberals tabled the bill, two key issues turned the support of the CMA and its provincial division, the B.C. Medical Association (BCMA), on its head.

The first issue concerned who would and who would not be covered by the state-run health plan. Doctors wanted the bill to focus narrowly on low-income earners and their dependants. Although the legislation promised coverage for low-wage earners, it left out the unemployed poor. The BCMA argued that doctors would "continue to carry this whole load of unpaid work" servicing the poor unless the unemployed were included.

While doctors understood that state payment for the poor would significantly boost their incomes, they asserted that the income ceilings used to determine a patient's eligibility for coverage were far too high. The CMA and its provincial division insisted that doctors must retain the ability to charge their higher earning patients more than the fees set in a state-run plan catering to the working poor. The doctors' organizations believed that the high ceilings would allow the government to "steal" patients who otherwise would pay whatever the doctor billed. The annual income ceilings originally proposed were reduced by 30 percent during the government's efforts to placate the medical profession.

The second issue was method of payment and the amount doctors would receive for each low-income patient. The proposed bill stipulated that general practitioners would be paid a set annual amount for each patient in their practice (i.e., capitation), while specialists would receive a separate payment for each act of service rendered, a method known as fee-for-service. In the BCMA's opinion, the capitation fees were too low and would condemn "the majority of medical men" to "economic slavery." In any event, the organization exclusively favoured fee-for-service. To make the issue even murkier, the capitation fees proposed by the government matched those recommended by the CMA, a position that contradicted the group's 1934 policy document, which rejected a uniform system of remuneration for physicians. In the end the CMA insisted that doctors – and only doctors – should decide how and how much they would be paid.

The B.C. legislation failed to meet these two demands as well as a host of others from the medical profession. In addition, B.C. doctors insisted that if the plan was to proceed within the tight financial constraints imposed by the Depression, either the number of medical services covered should be reduced or more money should be allocated to physician fees.

As plans to implement the health insurance scheme moved ahead, opposition mounted within B.C.'s business community. When the Royal Commission released its report in 1932, leading businessmen had urged the government to reject the recommendations for public health insurance, demanding instead a balanced budget and further spending restraints. The B.C. Manufacturers' Association, the Board of Trade, and the Chamber of Commerce vehemently opposed a payroll tax, charging that such a levy would give an unfair advantage to eastern competitors. They were joined in their opposition by property owners who feared that their property taxes would be increased to help pay for the plan.

Finally, insurance agencies made their voices heard. The Canadian

Life Insurance Officers' Association (CLIOA) generally supported B.C.'s efforts to insure the poor, although some of the association's more outspoken leaders were on record attacking any move towards a social — as opposed to a private — insurance model. But private insurers were in the process of solidifying a relationship with the CMA at the national level, and CLIOA's position on the B.C. plan seemed to reflect this agenda. CLIOA asserted that the plan lacked "equitable bases of remuneration for the medical profession" and would benefit from an "impartial review" by private-sector insurance experts.

Despite the opposition from both organized medicine and big business, the bill received royal assent on April 1, 1936. The government had strong public support when it announced the health plan would become operational one year later. But by this time the Liberals knew financing the plan, even in its modified form, would be difficult without federal assistance. As early as 1935 the B.C. government had tried to obtain a loan from Ottawa in order to finance the health scheme and other social programs, but it was turned down by Prime Minister R. B. Bennett, a Conservative. In October of that year, when the Mackenzie King Liberals took the reins of power in a national election, B.C.'s governing Liberals had high expectations that their federal comrades would help fund the program. But when the hopeful provincial hand was extended, it came back empty. The new federal government might have been Liberal, but it was in a fiscally conservative frame of mind.

The B.C. government was in trouble. In February 1937, just before public health insurance was to become a reality in British Columbia, the Vancouver Board of Trade and the BCMA cosponsored a protest meeting at the Hotel Georgia, attended by 400 people. With a near-unanimous show of hands, those in attendance denounced the health insurance plan. The Liberal government, heading into an election and stung by the bitterness of the medicare dispute, tried to bury the health insurance issue altogether, although a plebiscite on the question conducted during the campaign drew strong support. When the Liberals were returned to office in June 1937, they did not proclaim the legislation, consigning it, instead, to a limbo where it remained for nearly twenty years.

The doctors, meanwhile, moved to preempt any similar future initiatives by the government. In 1940 they established one of Canada's first physician-sponsored health-insurance plans, B.C. Medical Services Associated, which served as a model for doctors under the same threat in other provinces.

A burgeoning alliance

It was the coming together of the business community and the "medical men," combined with the weakening commitment of the Liberal government, that doomed public health insurance in British Columbia in 1937 despite substantial public support. The business community had openly campaigned against the legislation from the first day it was tabled and continued to apply pressure on the Liberal caucus in the legislature, and there were unconfirmed allegations that the CMA had allocated $10,000 to fund the B.C. medical profession's opposition to the bill.

While doctors and businessmen had their separate and distinct interests to protect in the debate, theirs was a marriage of convenience that would serve both groups well over the years. In the face of growing public interest in and support for government-sponsored insurance, any opposition to a plan that would so clearly benefit the majority of Canadians had to be carefully mounted. Depression-weary citizens had little trust in the corporate sector, so business needed to enlist a respected ally for the fight against public health insurance.

Many people identified doctors as advocates of medical relief for the poor in a number of municipalities during the 1930s. In some parts of Canada, doctors were joining the ranks of the poor themselves, notably in the Alberta and Saskatchewan dust bowls, while many others were critical of the choices forced upon their patients by poverty and the regressive policies of government. In addition, in the eyes of many patients, doctors had a saint-like status – selfless and hardworking, caring for and healing the most vulnerable. Doctors, therefore, were the perfect moral front for a business sector suffering from low levels of public esteem. For their part, business leaders could exert political muscle in a fight of overriding interest to the medical profession.

The British Columbia initiative provided organized medicine at both the provincial and national levels with its first practical test in politics. Doctors had successfully organized earlier in the century to ensure they held control of licensing and regulation of the medical profession. The CMA also was active in organizing against other professional groups, such as chiropractors, that were trying to gain a foothold in the field. But these were considered to be internal issues. Health insurance was the first "public interest" campaign organized medicine had involved itself in. And the fight in B.C. had shown the business community the value of acquiring doctors as allies in its fight against a public health insurance scheme that surely would redistribute tax dollars to the public – a direction they opposed. When Saskatchewan's CCF government moved to introduce a universal medical insurance program in 1959, organized medicine and the business community knew how to link arms to safeguard their private purses.

TWO

'A British Columbia and Saskatchewan Freak'

The unemployment crisis of the 1930s ended when Canada entered World War II and sent its Depression-idled youth to the battlefields of Europe. The impact of a gruelling decade of poverty, unemployment, and limited access to health services for most of the population was reflected in a 44 percent rejection rate due to poor health among the young men called up for selective service in Canada's armed forces. A similar percentage of people from the workforce that served on Canada's production lines (and that included a growing number of working women) was in less than perfect health as well. These figures shocked Canadians and reinforced the already compelling argument that health was an issue that affected all citizens individually and collectively.

Added to this gloomy picture were statistics that showed Canada ranked seventeenth among industrialized countries in infant mortality, with rates of between 38 and 80 deaths for every 1000 live births, depending on where one lived. Because access to hospital care was limited, approximately 3 to 5 women died in childbirth for every 1000 live births. Over 9800 Canadians died in 1940 alone from communicable diseases such as influenza, tuberculosis, diphtheria, measles, and whooping cough. Children and youth, especially in rural areas, were found to be in alarmingly poor health as well. In Manitoba in 1941, for example, 70 percent of those between thirteen and thirty years of age required some kind of medical attention. In each year between 1931 and 1941, an average of 15,000 Canadian children under one year of age died from preventable or controllable illnesses.

For the first time, Canadians were presented with statistical evidence that illustrated the dismal state of the public's health, and they were appalled. These factors, coupled with a decade of poverty and growing gaps between rich and poor, led the Canadian people to seek and demand alternatives. They had high expectations for a more equitable future, which included a strong safety net that would protect them and each succeeding generation from the cruelties and injustices they and their neighbours had had to endure throughout the previous decade.

A national health sytem

As early as 1939 the question of national health insurance was on the minds of several Members of Parliament who were keenly aware of the public mood. Soon after Canada entered the war, Ian Mackenzie, the minister of Pensions and National Health, urged Prime Minister Mackenzie King to respond positively to public sentiment favouring both unemployment insurance and "a national health system" that would cover both medical and hospital services. Mackenzie King favoured a postponement until peace had been secured in Europe. The country's resources, he said, would be pressed into service "until victory was won" and could not be spared for "social security matters."

In spite of Canada's wartime commitments and the prime minister's priorities, however, the Liberals inched forward. In early 1942 the federal Cabinet appointed an interdepartmental advisory committee on health insurance to draw up a blueprint for a national health program. Within a year this committee had drafted the first plans for a national health insurance scheme in Canada, but in 1945, when a national election was called, the Liberals had not implemented the program and the issue became a central one for all parties during the campaign. There was mounting anger among voters waiting impatiently for their demands for increased social spending to be met. In a letter to the prime minister, Ian Mackenzie warned that the unpopularity of the Liberals was due in part to the "rise of socialism all across Canada ... It was for years a British Columbia and Saskatchewan freak, but it is now definitely a national political menace." With his popularity in doubt, the CCF on his heels, and growing support among Canadians for a national hospital-medical insurance plan, the prime minister decided to heed the warnings of his health minister in word if not in deed.

During the national election campaign, all party platforms included a commitment to some kind of public health insurance scheme. The Liberals' was set out in vague policy statements presented by the prime minister. Mackenzie King's plan to proceed with a nationwide system of health insurance was intended to counter the CCF's call for a universal hospital and medical plan. But he made it clear the Liberals would not move ahead until they reached an agreement with the provinces about how such a plan would be administered and financed. Thus the ball was neatly pitched into the provinces' court in a well-practised federal manoeuvre.

On August 6, 1945, less than two months after the Liberals were reelected, the government convened the first Dominion-Provincial Conference to review proposals for post-war reconstruction in Canada. At the top of the agenda was health insurance. Mindful of recent public opinion polls showing 80 percent of Canadians supported a national health plan, and cautious about provincial jurisdictional claims, the federal government proposed a four-part strategy to bring about universal health insurance.

In the first step of the strategy, the government in Ottawa would allocate grants to each province to assist them in planning and organizing health insurance benefits. The second part of the strategy would be introduced in stages: since no one knew how much money would be required to establish full comprehensive coverage, Ottawa would pay for 20 percent of the estimated costs for general practitioner services, hospital care, and visiting nursing services. After three years the federal government would increase its contribution to 50 percent of the actual cost of each benefit included in provincial health insurance plans. Later still, other medical services (for example, specialists and other health professionals), private nursing care, drugs, and laboratory services would be included in provincial health insurance schemes, with Ottawa's contribution reaching 60 percent of the cost of each benefit. The third point in the strategy involved a system of health grants for provinces to implement specific measures such as programs to treat patients with mental health problems or tuberculosis, while the fourth and final part would extend federal assistance for hospital construction.

In exchange for substantial federal support for health and other social services, the provinces would have to agree that the collection of personal income, corporation, and inheritance taxes would revert back to Ottawa exclusively. (The collection of these tax revenues had been shared between federal and provincial governments under wartime emergency arrangements.) In addition, minimum standards for health and social services would have to be maintained in each province and each province would have to commit to the plan for a trial period of three years.

While the four western provinces supported the federal government's strategy, the other six, led by Ontario, were less enthusiastic. Discussions continued until May 1946, when the Dominion-Provincial Conference collapsed in acrimony about jurisdiction, tax collection, money, and cost sharing without having reached agreement.

A waiting game then ensued: the provinces waited for Ottawa to initiate legislation establishing a cost-sharing formula between the two levels of government; Ottawa waited for the provinces to commit themselves to its proposed blueprint.

While many in the Mackenzie King government occupied themselves with the socialistic "British Columbia and Saskatchewan freak" that threatened to sweep the land, investor-owned insurance companies and nonprofit physician-sponsored insurance plans were busy reconciling their differences and forming a mutually beneficial alliance to fight the battle against "socialized medicine" and its perceived threat to free enterprise.

The rise of nonprofit and commercial health insurance

When debates about public health programs emerged with renewed vigour during the Great Depression, life insurance had been around almost a hundred years, but commercial health insurance was still rare in Canada. It wasn't until World War II and after, when Canadian incomes increased during the post-war period, that private or "investor-owned" insurance companies entered the health field to any significant degree.

Up to that point, Canadian health insurance had evolved in two parallel streams during the twentieth century. Insurance to cover hospital services was established to meet the needs of injured workers and others who required emergency care. By pooling their own resources – and with support from religious orders, unions, agricultural organizations, and employers – workers and farmers established insurance cooperatives that would pay for a hospital bed and related services such as laboratory tests, X-rays, surgery, and nursing care received when a member of the cooperative was ill or convalescing. Hospital insurance did not cover medical services offered in the doctor's office (for example, physical or eye examinations, vaccinations, or stitches), so separate but parallel health insurance plans emerged in many parts of the country.

The growing interest in public health insurance, and the emergence of consumer insurance cooperatives covering both hospital and physician services, led the medical profession to develop its own plans aimed at subsidizing low-income earners who otherwise could not afford medical services. Doctors hoped that by sponsoring insurance coverage for physician services they would achieve a number of goals. First, by providing an affordable and nonprofit insurance scheme to subsidize the working poor, they could establish two tiers: one for low-income earners who would receive services specified on the physician plan; another for patients who could afford to pay their own fees or could afford coverage from private insurers, and who could be charged full market rates. In this way, doctors could exercise more control over their incomes and, importantly, their medical practices without outside interference.

In addition, doctors hoped that by expanding access to physician services they would dampen enthusiasm for government-sponsored health insurance. Several provinces had established commissions of inquiry to look at public health schemes during the 1930s. The experience of doctors in British Columbia in 1935 to 1937 had convinced many of their colleagues across the country that so-called "voluntary" insurance sponsored by the medical profession – as opposed to universal, state-sponsored plans – might be the answer. The use of the terms "voluntary" to describe physician-sponsored health insurance and "compulsory" to characterize tax-supported government plans was a tactic laced with ideology. Who, after all, would support compulsion over freedom and choice?

The first experiment with a physician-sponsored insurance scheme occurred in 1939 in Windsor, Ontario, where the local medical society had obtained support from the Ontario Medical Association (OMA) for the subsidy idea. The OMA's new president, Dr. W. K. Colbeck, had greeted the proposal with a strong endorsement. "If we do not socialize ourselves and develop the proper technique of service," Colbeck said, "governments will be forced to try their hand." Soon after, Toronto doctors set up Associated Medical Services (AMS) for the Ontario Civil Service Association. Founded by Dr. J. A. Hannah, a leading opponent of "state medicine," the AMS boasted offices in ten centres around the province by 1942. By sponsoring health insurance, said Dr. Hannah, "the medical profession will assume leadership in securing public co-operation and thus see to it that Government regulation shall be only such minimum as will enable us to exercise proper control over ourselves and the public."

Doctors across the country jumped on the bandwagon so "that medical coverage can be obtained at a satisfactory premium without [government] interference and regulation." By the late 1940s, most provinces had physician-sponsored, prepaid, medical insurance schemes that targeted indigents and low-income workers whose earnings fell below physician-specified income ceilings. Patients in high-risk categories, who often were rejected by the growing for-profit insurance industry, were accepted by many doctors' plans, as were the poor.

The prepaid, or voluntary, insurance plans were operated on a non-profit basis, a characteristic that distinguished them from their commercial competitors. The plans offered what were called "service contracts," in which the doctor billed the plan directly instead of billing his or her low-income patients. The plans contracted with the doctor, whose fees adhered to a schedule agreed to by the plan and the provincial medical association. Extra billing (or additional charges above the fee schedule) was prohibited in the service contract, but the arrangement enabled doctors to bill their higher income patients on a sliding scale – the higher the income, the higher the physician's fee.

The physician-sponsored plans, with the advantage of the service contract, proved to be very popular. Consequently, plan administrators began to remove the income limits to enable broader coverage. As enrollment increased among higher income subscribers, doctors began to demand the right to extra-bill their wealthier patients above the plan's fee schedule. Nonetheless, the plans found favour among most physicians, who saw their average net incomes rise by over 150 percent from 1941 to 1949, with a further 71 percent increase over the next ten years. Prepaid insurance plans also forced doctors to establish a uniform rate or tariff for each item of service. These rates would apply regardless of who the payer was – patient or government, physician-sponsored or commercial insurer. While medical fee schedules imposed uniform rates on doctors (much to their dismay), they also standardized fee-for-service as the method of payment, enabling doctors to bill, and eventually to extra-bill, for each service rendered.

Physician-sponsored plans were not the only nonprofit private insurers in Canada. By 1934 there were twenty-seven hospital-based prepayment plans successfully operating in six provinces across the country. Five years later, Winnipeg hospitals and community groups joined together to form the country's first Blue Cross plan. The plan was unique in that it was sponsored by the Central Council of Social Agencies in Winnipeg, with a board of directors composed of representatives from labour, business, farmers, and rural municipalities. By

1957 Manitoba Blue Cross had enrolled 46 percent of the province's population, making it the largest such plan in Canada. Its remarkable success spawned a cross-Canada movement, an indication of the limitations in insurance schemes covering medical services alone.

In Ontario, the Hospital Association established a Blue Cross plan in 1941 for commercial and industrial groups, but excluded rural subscribers. By 1958 Blue Cross represented 39 percent of the Ontario population, making it the sixth largest Blue Cross plan in North America. During the 1940s B.C., Québec, Alberta, and the Maritimes all had hospital-sponsored Blue Cross plans. The Québec and Maritime plans provided medical benefits in addition to hospital services. Over 3 million people were insured by Blue Cross plans across the country by 1952, out of a total of 5.5 million covered by hospital insurance.[1]

By 1961, 53 percent of Canadians were enrolled in medical or hospital insurance plans (up from 6 percent in 1943), divided almost equally between the nonprofit prepayment plans and more than a hundred commercial insurers. Competition between the two was intense, despite the not-for-profit principles that guided (somewhat loosely) the physician- and hospital-sponsored plans. It was usual for Blue Cross and physician-sponsored plans to keep up to 15 percent of premiums collected to offset administrative overhead. But during standing committee hearings on hospital insurance in Ontario in 1956, provincial CCF leader Donald MacDonald revealed that benefit payouts to customers of the four leading commercial insurers ranged from 39 to 61 percent of the total premiums collected. The difference (minus administration) went to shareholders and investors.

One reason for the success of the commercial insurers lay in the profile of their clientele and the structure of the coverage they offered. Nonprofit insurers such as Blue Cross charged the same rate for the provision of hospital services regardless of the type of service provided or the subscriber's income, while physician-sponsored plans covered services offered in the doctor's office but varied the subscription fee depending on the patient's income. Most commercial insurers subjected individuals to a "risk classification" process, identifying characteristics such as age, sex, health, occupation, and hobbies that would determine premium rates – or would disqualify the applicant altogether – and they preferred younger, healthier men who required fewer services. Commercial insurers identified a range of conditions as "risky," including the condition of being female, being too old, too young, too sick, too disabled, or of being pregnant, chronically ill, unemployed, or employed in a hazardous industry. Insurance premiums for individuals were often prohibitively high, in sharp contrast to many nonprofit plans, but commercial companies could offer much lower group rates to employers with a healthy workforce.

Commercial and nonprofit insurers both offered individual and group health plans, but most premium income came from the latter. The two groups competed for business from employers who purchased group plans and could negotiate group rates with the insurer. Commercial insurers did not require medical examinations for those covered under such a policy, but they did rate the risks associated with a workforce profile and charged accordingly. Employers whose workforce was young, healthy, and male were charged lower premiums than those who employed women or older workers, or who were engaged in a less healthy line of business. Under group plans, workers normally would pay part of the premium, called a co-payment. The plans seldom covered the entire fee charged for a medical or hospital service, so employees were required to pay a portion of the bill, known as a deductible. The exclusion of spouses and children from group health plans also lowered the employer's premium rates, but intentionally or not, it meant that women and children in Canada suffered from discriminatory policies that raised the financial risks associated with illness among an already vulnerable population.

Commercial or investor-owned insurance companies enjoyed good relations with the business sector, with which they shared a common, and conservative, political outlook. Their relations with the medical profession, on the other hand, were often tense. Until the 1960s the two groups disagreed about whether the standard 30 percent "commission" insurers built into their premium charges for the sale of medical services was legitimate. Doctors also rejected the intervention of a third party between them and their patients, since it represented a threat to physician autonomy. These differences gave the competition between investor-owned and nonprofit insurers an ideological flavour that at times was enunciated with sanctimonious righteousness by doctors whose net incomes had benefitted enormously from the growth of the insurance industry.

As doctors' incomes continued to rise, so too did their tolerance for profit making in medicine. Many doctors became increasingly critical of the nonprofit plans because of continuing restrictions imposed on extra billing. Investor-owned companies attempted (often successfully) to lure doctors away from the nonprofits with what was called indemnity insurance – a plan that allowed doctors to set their own fees and bill the patient directly for services rendered. Under the indemnity plans, patients would pay the doctor and submit the paid invoice to the insurer who would "indemnify" – or reimburse – the cost in whole or, more likely, in part. In addition to the deductible on indemnity plans, patients often had to pay doctors an extra-billing charge, so physicians usually made more money from their business with commercial insurers. Finally, a patient covered by an indemnity plan was only entitled to the procedures specified in his or her particular plan. If other services were rendered, patients paid directly out of pocket or, alternatively, paid a higher premium for broader coverage.

Since group and individual health policies were renewed annually, competition between commercial and nonprofit insurers was unrelenting. After World War II, commercial carriers began offering a variety of packages to subscribers. More costly options such as "major medical" or extended health, insurers said, would "enhance" health coverage for those with risky illnesses or chronic conditions. Supplementary benefits were optional and covered "extras" such as physiotherapy and health services supplied by professionals other than physicians. With the introduction of medicare, extended or supplementary health insurance would come to include professional, dental, psychological, and other health services not included on the public health insurance plan. Coverage for drugs, certain types of medical or drug delivery aids, and unlimited ambulance transport also would fall to the private insurance market. In spite of this growing – and often confusing – number of options, a majority of subscribers were covered inadequately.

The establishment of nonprofit hospital- or physician-sponsored plans during the 1930s and 1940s, begun mainly to avert the threat of socialized medicine, enabled many individuals excluded by commercial insurers to obtain minimal protection. Commercial insurers concentrated on the employed, whose coverage on group health plans was sponsored – and paid for – by employers, and on "insurable" individuals. As Dr. Jason A. Hannah, a pioneer of the physician-sponsored prepayment movement, put it, prior to World War II commercial health insurance often "was available only if the individual was employed and remained 'insurable'. Women and children, not being gainfully employed, were considered uninsurable. Also, those suffering from chronic illness, or beyond their sixty-fifth birthday were considered uninsurable, as were those who contracted conditions which might have a deleterious affect on health, ... although they might have been paying premiums for years without drawing any benefits."

Since policies were renewable annually, Hannah said, individuals who developed a chronic condition "became uninsurable and were dropped at the end of the policy year in which the condition appeared." Those who were unable to work because of an illness would still be required to pay premiums for medical coverage if they continued to meet the insurer's risk criteria. If they did pass the risk assessment but could not afford the premiums, they lost their medical coverage and their access to medical care – a kind of double jeopardy. These practices created fertile ground for nonprofit carriers and by 1961 many of the 263 organizations in Canada licensed to provide health insurance were classified outside of the commercial sector.

Although just over half of Canadians had medical insurance by the mid-1950s, there was by no means equitable distribution of health, health services, or the financial burdens associated with the cost of care among all the population. A report compiled by the Dominion Bureau of Statistics showed that during 1950-1951, people with the highest incomes obtained the lion's share of health-care services even though the people with the lowest income experienced more illness more often. In addition, the severity of illness was greater amongst low-income groups, particularly among men, who showed higher rates of tuberculosis and accidents requiring hospitalization. Based on a comprehensive sickness survey of 40,000 households, the report offered statistical evidence to support what was already widely known: that poor people were sick more often and that there was a direct relationship between level of income and the volume of health services received.

First steps to medicare

There were no hospital-sponsored Blue Cross plans in Saskatchewan or B.C. This was because in 1947 the CCF government in Saskatchewan, tired of waiting for Ottawa to move forward on national health insurance, took a first tentative step towards medicare. Premier Tommy Douglas was determined that if he had anything to do with it, "people would be able to get health services just as they are able to get educational services, as an inalienable right of being a citizen." It was widely recognized that provinces would be unable to support the full-blown health insurance scheme Ottawa contemplated without substantial financial input from the federal government. Under Douglas's leadership, therefore, the Saskatchewan government introduced universal hospital insurance. The British Columbia government followed its lead in 1949. This was an important breakthrough in the stalemate over national health insurance.

Saskatchewan's hospital plan, backed by near-unanimous public support, was structured to meet criteria sketched out in Ottawa's 1945 blueprint so that when federal contributions were forthcoming, the province would qualify to receive them. When this happened, Saskatchewan would be well positioned to introduce North America's first system of universal health insurance covering both physician and hospital services. Hospital insurance was not quite the full and universal health-care system the CCF wanted, but the province would have to wait until federal contributions became available before it could proceed.

These developments in the two "freak" provinces stirred unease among the nation's medical profession. Doctors began laying the groundwork for a united front to oppose a government-sponsored plan for physician services, an event that was viewed as inevitable if hospital insurance caught on. In 1951 the CMA brought all of the provincially based, doctor-run plans under the umbrella of the Trans-Canada Medical Plan (TCMP). Two years later, hospital-sponsored insurers in Québec and the Maritimes were accepted as members, despite the fact that physicians neither sponsored nor controlled the plans. Within ten years, this consortium provided hospital and/or physician insurance to almost 25 percent of the population across the country.

The rationale for founding the TCMP was heavily influenced by the CMA's political agenda. "We require a corporation which can function all over Canada and which could not be ignored by any government," said the chair of the CMA's influential economics committee, and the provincial divisions were in agreement. A confidential paper presented to a 1951 meeting of officials from Saskatchewan's two doctor-run medical insurers explained that the prepayment plans provided "a sound method" for residents to prepay their health needs, "thereby eliminating a demand for government-sponsored, compulsory health insurance." With public opinion 80 percent in favour of a national public health program, it "was both urgent and desirable" to establish physician-sponsored, prepaid medical services. If proof was needed, one could look at British Columbia where "the threat of a compulsory plan in ... 1935 [had] brought the profession in that province to its feet in one organized group to sponsor BC Medical Services Associated" five years later. By 1960, insurers were organized into two syndicates: nonprofit physician and hospital plans under the TCMP umbrella; for-profit commercial operators united in the Canadian Health Insurance Association founded the year before.

With continued public interest in a national health plan, and growing provincial interest spurred by the experiments with hospital insurance in B.C. and Saskatchewan, the federal government tabled proposals for a national hospital insurance program late in 1955.

The Hospital Insurance and Diagnostic Services (HIDS) Act, passed on April 10, 1957, was a turning point in Canada's medicare history for a number of reasons. First, the federal Liberals had finally moved towards a policy goal enunciated during a party convention in 1919 (and which was subsequently buried for nearly forty years). It was a step taken reluctantly by Prime Minister Louis St. Laurent, but one that Health Minister Paul Martin Sr. was both personally and politically committed to.

Second, the years between 1919 and 1958 (when HIDS was fully operational) were marked by heated and sometimes bitter debates about public health insurance and the costs associated with such a program. During this period, business and physician groups with a vested interest in private health care and low corporate tax rates had emerged and formed powerful alliances, making support for a full program of insured hospital and physician services more of a political gamble for politicians.

Finally, and perhaps most importantly, the HIDS Act allocated federal funds to provinces with a universal hospital insurance program as long as the program met national criteria for "uniform terms and conditions."

Not surprisingly, the HIDS Act was opposed by the CMA, the commercial insurance industry, the Canadian Hospital Association (CHA), and the Canadian Chamber of Commerce. In 1956 the CMA warned that the legislation was a first move towards full, universal, government-controlled health care in Canada – a move that most people supported but that most doctors did not. If hospital insurance was introduced, the CMA charged, then socialized medicine could not be far behind.

Private insurers called public hospital insurance a "Trojan Horse" that would "destroy ... freedom of choice" because people – in particular healthy high income earners, the industry's target consumer – would no longer be able to choose from among dozens of insurance policies and instead would be forced onto public health plans. "Compulsory health insurance," the industry concluded, "cannot be separated from state medicine and socialism." The Chamber of Commerce also decried "state medicine" and the abuses it claimed were inevitable by "persons demanding treatment as a right for imaginary ills or illnesses."

Though the CHA said that a "National Health Program" excluding nursing homes, home-care programs, and homes for the elderly would place unmanageable pressures on the nation's hospitals, it did not advocate an expanded hospital plan. Instead, along with the CMA and the insurance industry, hospitals advocated government subsidies to enable the poor to subscribe to private health plans.

In their separate submissions to the parliamentary committee on national hospital insurance, the medical profession, hospital administrators, private insurers, and the business community coalesced around the position that would ally them in their later opposition to medicare. Each group had a direct interest in protecting private health insurance, whether it was for-profit or nonprofit. Although the doctor-run plans and hospital-sponsored Blue Cross competed for subscribers with Canada's commercial insurers, they cast aside their rivalries to stand together against the threat emanating from a public plan that would surely eliminate all of them from the health insurance field altogether.

While these groups vigorously resisted state-sponsored hospital insurance, they were not opposed to the idea that public funds could be used to enroll the uninsurable in private plans. This, in fact, was the key proposal made to the parliamentary committee by the CMA, the CHA, the Chamber of Commerce, and CLIOA (CHIA's forerunner). Low-income earners and those in high-risk categories, they maintained, should receive a subsidy from their provincial governments so they could purchase, if they chose, a health insurance policy from either a commercial company or one of the TCMP plans.

Despite criticism of the bill, the HIDS Act passed with unanimous consent in the House of Commons. When the legislation was enacted, five provinces – British Columbia, Alberta, Saskatchewan, Ontario, and Newfoundland – had agreed to sign on. Five days after the Senate gave its stamp of approval, Prince Edward Island announced it would sign an agreement with Ottawa to provide universal hospital insurance as well. By 1961, all ten provinces were eligible for federal cost sharing to provide universal hospital insurance.

The Liberals, who had counted on the legislation to help them win the next election, were narrowly defeated by the Progressive Conservatives in June 1957. John Diefenbaker formed a government committed to the HIDS Act (with some minor amendments) and announced the plan would be fully operational on July 1, 1958. Less than ten months later, with over $13 million coming into the province under the federal-provincial cost-sharing arrangement for hospital insurance, Saskatchewan Premier Tommy Douglas announced that his government would introduce a universal health insurance plan.

The battle in Saskatchewan

When Douglas announced the government's plan for a "complete transfer of medicare expenditures from the private to the public sector," the reaction of the province's physicians, newspapers, and business community was immediate, ferocious, and uniformly hostile to the government's proposals. The public, on the other hand, had expected the CCF government to fulfill its longstanding promise to introduce universal public hospital and physician insurance, and were well disposed towards the idea.

Although Saskatchewan residents could obtain health insurance from one of two prepayment plans or through a commercial carrier, one third of the population had no protection of any kind. Many found medical insurance too costly while others were covered inadequately. Even with insurance, direct payments by patients – the portion of the physician's fee that was extra-billed – accounted for over 45 percent of doctors' total earnings, pushing physician incomes in Saskatchewan higher than anywhere else in the country. The goal of the Saskatchewan CCF and of the public generally was to ensure that all residents could obtain health services without financial or other barriers restricting access.

The goal of the doctors was to retain the status quo, and they had a formidable tool in their fight – the Saskatchewan College of Physicians and Surgeons (SCPS). In most provinces the CMA's provincial divisions were voluntary associations responsible for developing fee-for-service schedules, negotiating the terms of service contracts with physician-sponsored or commercial insurance plans, and carrying out public relations and political lobbying. Physician colleges, on the other hand, were responsible for licensing practitioners and regulating their activities, and membership was not an option: those who did not join did not practise. The SCPS, however, played a dual role. Not only was it

Saskatchewan's regulatory body for the medical profession, it also acted as the CMA's political arm in the province. Membership in the SCPS was compulsory and universal: any doctor practising in Saskatchewan was required to join. As a result, doctors in favour of the government's plan for tax-supported and universal public health insurance feared that their licences would be cancelled if they publicly endorsed the plan. Consequently the voices of pro-medicare physicians in Saskatchewan were silenced.

Until 1950 the Saskatchewan medical profession had been on record supporting "state-aided health insurance." But the growth and popularity of the physician-sponsored prepayment plans had persuaded many doctors in Saskatchewan that the kind of state aid proposed by the CCF was unnecessary and, perhaps more to the point, would seriously erode the almost total control they exercised over the public's use of medical services. In 1959 the SCPS had formally reversed its position, rejecting a "compulsory, government-controlled, province-wide medical care plan" in favour of "the extension of health and accident benefits through indemnity and service plans."

This shift in the profession's support for public health insurance was, perhaps, understandable. But Saskatchewan physicians' abandonment of their staunch loyalty to the TCMP service contract model was surprising and reflected the growing ideological alliance between doctors and the commercial insurance industry. The rapid expansion of the commercial insurance market had convinced the CMA and its provincial divisions that they could no longer afford to keep their increasingly powerful for-profit rivals at a distance. For their part, commercial insurers wanted to strengthen their ties with the medical profession, arguing that it was in the interest of doctors to support what was called a "multiple carrier approach" that gave customers the choice between for-profit and nonprofit (but not, of course, between public and private) insurance carriers.

During the pitched battle that followed Douglas's momentous announcement, the SCPS solidified its links with the business community, the opposition Liberals, drug companies, the Dental Association, and the Sifton family newspaper chain (which controlled the Regina *Leader-Post* and the Saskatoon *Star-Phoenix*). Together, these groups engineered an intense campaign against the provincial government's health plan. The campaign peaked with a doctors' strike that began on July 1, 1962, the day the plan came into effect, and lasted for twenty-three days.

The Saskatchewan press, which referred to July 1 as "the day when Freedom died," was unrelenting in its attacks both on medicare and the CCF. At cocktail parties hosted by the business community for the national and international press that descended on the province to witness the strike, the new alliance zeroed in on what it saw as the main issue: socialism and the destruction of the economy versus free enterprise. The SCPS and the Chamber of Commerce, which accused the government of trying to impose a state monopoly over health care, reiterated their by now familiar demand that low-income subscribers be given a subsidy to purchase private or prepaid health insurance.

The CMA at the national level did not sit idly by as tensions escalated in the prairie province. Its horror of public health insurance convinced it that Saskatchewan's doctors were on the frontlines of the battle against socialized medicine, in defence of the free enterprise system. The CMA ended up contributing nearly $100,000 to Saskatchewan's doctors to aid the fight against the CCF's health insurance proposal, adding to the $60,000 the College had raised through a membership levy. The CMA also coordinated doctors nationwide in support of their Saskatchewan colleagues.

Doctors, along with their business allies, pulled out all the stops during the strike, launching a racist attack on the foreign physicians who had gone to Saskatchewan at the invitation of the government to provide medical services. Patients who were female and Catholic were warned that they would be forced to violate church doctrines on birth control if the government took charge of health care. The SCPS said doctors would leave the province if medicare was introduced, a threat that resonated in rural Saskatchewan where doctors were few and far between. But despite the tactics of an organized and well-financed anti-medicare alliance, the public – which had been sympathetic at the peak of the campaign – began to waver in its support. Physicians had rejected every concession from the government and had taken unprecedented action to support what appeared now to be a self-serving position rather than one defending high standards of care. On July 23 a "treaty" was signed between the SCPS and the embattled government. It would greatly influence the discussions now underway at the national level about the future of Canada's health-care system.

This agreement included an acceptance by the SCPS that medicare in Saskatchewan would be universal and compulsory and that the government would be the sole collector of revenues and disburser of payments. For its part, the government agreed that the doctors' prepayment plans would be maintained and would act as "billing and payment conduits" for physicians who did not want a relationship with the new Medical Care Insurance Commission (MCIC), which was to act at arm's length from the government.

To secure the signature of the SCPS, the government was forced to introduce legislation indicating it would not establish a medical service with full-time, salaried practitioners. Finally, and again at the insistence of the SCPS, all references to the maintenance and improvement of quality care were removed from the Medical Care Insurance Act, and the MCIC was reduced to a collection and payment agency rather than a public administrator of the health-care system.

In January 1962 in its presentation to the Royal Commission on Health Services (see chapter 3), the government of Saskatchewan said, "Health services must be viewed as public services which can be best planned, organized, administered and financed by government." This position was in keeping with the vision of the CCF, but the concessions forced from the government by the medical profession, the business community, commercial insurers, and the Sifton family press resulted in services that were financed by government but that remained "planned, organized [and] administered" by the private and, at the time, mainly nonprofit sector. It was an important and defining moment in Canada's slow progress toward a national health program, setting a precedent that would be followed in federal legislation five years later.

Despite the concessions, however, the people of Saskatchewan, with a committed and farsighted provincial government, had achieved what no one else in the country had at that time. Medicare in the prairie province fired the imagination of Canadians and made the idea of a full, national, public health program a tangible thing, a realistic goal rather than a dream. Alone among Canadians – alone, in fact, on the continent – Saskatchewan residents could not be denied access to medical services because of an existing illness or condition, because they could not afford them, or because they were too old or were members of a "poor risk" group.

Commercial insurers, temporarily abandoned by their medical allies in the final hours of the conflict, were no longer able to offer health insurance in Saskatchewan because their system of deductibles, exclusions, and age restrictions precluded the principle of universality.

Physicians, on the other hand, fared very well. Doctors' incomes in the province increased by nearly 40 percent from 1960 to 1963, putting their annual earnings $3400 above the national average. While the SCPS vowed to continue its fight against socialized medicine, when its Liberal allies came to power in the 1964 provincial election there was little appetite to reverse direction, especially given the strong support for the medicare program among the public.

THREE

The Fight
For National
Medical Insurance

Though the insurance industry, the business community, and the Canadian Medical Association had viewed events in Saskatchewan with growing horror, they had not been absent from the national scene during this period. A 1960 Gallup poll showed that support among Canadians for a government-sponsored medicare program remained very high. Alarmed by the developments in Saskatchewan and dismayed at the continuing support for a state-run plan, the CMA wrote to Prime Minister John Diefenbaker urging a public debate on medicare outside the "hectic arena of political controversy." A Royal Commission was needed, said the CMA, to "[assess] the health needs and resources of Canada with a view to recommending methods of ensuring the highest standards of health care for all Canadians."

Nine days later, Diefenbaker announced a federal inquiry would be conducted. Within six months he had appointed all of the commissioners, and the Royal Commission on Health Services, headed by Emmett Hall, chief justice of Saskatchewan, began its deliberations. The timing coincided with the escalation of events in Saskatchewan and the establishment of a political and ideological alliance between the CMA and the newly founded Canadian Health Insurance Association (CHIA), representing 120 companies. Many physicians involved in the prepayment plans viewed the overtures from commercial carriers with suspicion and feared public resentment about what might appear as a "gang up" by the insurance industry. The CMA, however, suffered no such discomfort, and in 1961, commercial carriers and the TCMP (at the urging of the CMA) set up the Canadian Conference on Health Care. The Conference vowed to defeat any attempts to establish government health insurance, but endorsed the government-subsidy-for-the-poor idea. It called for such subsidies to be channelled to "multiple insurance organizations," either of the for-profit variety or of the nonprofit, physician-sponsored kind. The CMA and CHIA began collaborating on their submissions to the Hall Commission, which by the fall of 1961 had commenced hearings that doctors and private insurers feared could lead to increased demand for a national health insurance scheme – of the public kind.

The CHIA and the CMA focussed considerable energy in three directions, all of which were designed to protect private insurers and, by extension, private fee-for-service physician care in Canada. The first priority was to expand insurance coverage to a larger number of people and to broaden the list of services provided under private plans, which would have the added advantage of increasing premium revenues. In order to more effectively argue the benefits of private insurance coverage, the CMA and CHIA had to demonstrate that a growing number of people were able and willing to enroll in private plans, whether physician-sponsored or for-profit. A vigorous recruitment drive was underway by the early 1960s, and the number of insured Canadians continued to grow. In 1965, out of a population of over 18 million, some 5.6 million people were enrolled in TCMP plans across the country while another 5 million were covered by investor-owned insurance companies. But 7.5 million Canadians were without medical insurance of any kind, and of those who were enrolled in a plan, coverage often was inadequate and premiums and deductibles were very high.

The second priority was to preempt any further provincial initiatives to introduce a program of medicare such as Saskatchewan was then attempting to do. To this end the CHIA and CMA mounted an intensive lobby of provincial governments to convince them of the merits of the subsidy alternative. In 1963 they succeeded in Alberta, where the government introduced a plan to provide subsidies to assist low-income individuals and "medical indigents" enrolled in one of more than thirty private insurance carriers or in the profession-sponsored Medical Services (Alberta) Incorporated (MSAI). The government also set up a coordinating body – composed of the health minister, the Alberta College of Physicians and Surgeons, the CHIA, and MSAI – to administer the plan. Dubbed "Manningcare," after Premier Ernest Manning, the plan was widely criticized in Alberta because the premiums established in the legislation were higher than the premiums charged before the plan was introduced. In other words, the government had given private insurers a green light to raise the amount they charged subscribers. This placed insurance premium rates beyond the financial reach of a growing number of Albertans and increased the amount of revenue available to insurers and doctors under the subsidy program. Both the CMA and CHIA were ecstatic. Of the 1.1 million people insured in Alberta by March 1964, 300,000 qualified for a subsidy, but only 150,000 had applied. The remaining 150,000 chose to forego the humiliation of the means test.

After their victory in Alberta, the CMA-CHIA alliance turned its attention to British Columbia and Ontario. In April 1963 Ontario's Conservative government introduced medicare legislation to subsidize individuals on private or prepayment insurance plans. The legislation also established two types of service contracts, one at lower premium rates but requiring deductibles and co-payments from subscribers. The NDP and the Liberal Party of Ontario attacked the government for "leaning over backwards to be of assistance to the insurance companies." In response to mounting criticism from labour, the public, and media, the Conservative government retreated, setting up a committee to study the medicare question. In January 1966 it reintroduced the bill with amendments. The government would establish the Ontario Medical Services Insurance Plan (OMSIP) to insure high-risk groups and low-income earners, whose eligibility would be determined using income tax thresholds developed jointly by the CMA and CHIA. Again, the medical profession and the insurance industry were jubilant.

British Columbia, which for twenty-five years had maintained but not implemented its law on public health insurance, established the B.C. Medical Plan (BCMP) in 1965 to insure individuals who could not afford the premiums for private medical coverage, either because they were poor or because they were a "poor risk." This plan, reportedly developed over a series of dinner meetings between Premier W. A. C. Bennett and Dr. Peter Banks, head of the BCMA, ensured that private carriers and the doctor-sponsored MSA-BC would continue to operate without having to worry about the commercially uninsurable. Whereas Alberta subsidized low-income individuals' enrollment in private plans, BCMP and OMSIP assumed responsibility for those residents who fell below the income threshold or who would pose a daunting risk for the insurance industry.

The CMA-CHIA strategy focussing on provincial governments was developed in part because of the uncertainty surrounding the question of jurisdiction over health care. The terms of reference given the Hall Commission in June 1961 included an instruction that the commissioners "recommend such measures, consistent with the constitutional division of legislative powers in Canada, as the Commissioners believe will ensure that the best possible health care is available to all Canadians." But in the twenty-five years since the Royal Commission on Dominion-Provincial Relations, the constitutional wrangles over what role the federal government should and could play in health care had not been resolved. The CMA and its private insurance partners hoped that provinces with medical care insurance legislation in place would defend their constitutional prerogatives against any attempt by Ottawa to impose a national medicare plan.

The third direction in which the CMA-CHIA alliance expended its considerable energy and resources was the Royal Commission hearings, begun in the autumn of 1961 in the Maritimes. In their submissions to the Hall Commission, both the CMA and the CHIA pushed the idea of subsidies and the free market. Some 30 presentations out of 406 made to the commission supported the subsidy model. These came from the CMA and its ten provincial divisions, the Trans-Canada Medical Plan, chambers of commerce, and the private insurance industry.

The Hall Commission report

The report of the Hall Commission, released on June 19, 1964, was – and is, thirty-five years later – a compelling presentation of every aspect of Canada's health-care sector at the time and of the health status of Canadians. The commissioners conducted hearings across the country and received over 400 submissions from individuals and organizations, the majority of whom supported a government-sponsored health program. In addition, they spent a portion of their time studying the financing structures used in the health systems of Europe and the United States before writing their own recommendations for Canada.

In the first pages of the report, the commissioners argued that the expanding public interest in health grew out of Canadians' own history of community-based measures implemented to counter the epidemics over the previous century, including influenza and tuberculosis in the 1910s and 1920s. This tendency had deepened because of a growing "humanitarian concern for our fellows [in which] we recognize that the well-being and happiness of society is simply the sum total of the well-being and happiness of its individual members."

This humanitarianism was reinforced by the shock Canadians felt when, on the verge of World War II, they learned of some of the consequences of the country's neglect during the Great Depression. "The most dramatic evidence was the rejection rates of armed services recruits in World War II. With the nation in peril, dependent upon its healthy man- and woman-power for survival, the price we were paying for our past lack of adequate health resources and services was glaringly apparent."

An equal shock came with the release of the Sickness Survey in 1951, which "showed the appalling social and economic cost to Canada of ill-health" and the "failure to make available to all Canadian citizens the standard of health service we know how to provide." In addition to lost production (which in 1961 was estimated to be 52.7 million person-days), the report said, "many of our so-called 'welfare' expenditures are the end result of illness, disability, and premature death."

The commissioners reminded Canadians of their government's signature on the Charter of the World Health Organization, whose preamble declared: "The enjoyment of the highest attainable standard of health is one of the fundamental rights of every human being without distinction of race, religion, political belief, economic or social condition." It was essential, the commissioners stated, to use what Winston Churchill described as "the application of averages for the relief of millions" because though many Canadians who could afford to do so had "availed themselves of the insurance mechanism," less than half the population was reasonably protected from the financial consequences associated with illness and disease.

In their report for the Canadian government, the commissioners described "three related though basically different approaches" to the question of how to provide and pay for health services that were presented in the submissions they received. The nonprofit and for-profit private "insurance approach," was supported mainly by the insurance industry and the CMA. The medical profession and its sponsored health plans proposed the private, doctor-controlled "prepayment approach." The "health services approach," a tax-based, public system similar to England's, was supported by what the commissioners referred to as "consumer groups."

The insurance approach, the commissioners explained, was not "concerned principally with the supply of health resources." Although they did not comment on what private insurers were primarily concerned with, it was clear that maintaining healthy profit margins (as opposed to healthy populations) was high on the list of the industry's priorities and that complex strategies had been developed to meet this goal. One strategy was to divide Canadians into two groups: the insurable and the uninsurable. The insurable were divided again into two more groups, according to the Royal Commission: "those who can pay the necessary premiums from their own resources, and ... those who cannot pay all or any part of the premiums and who must, therefore, be subsidized, presumably by government."

In 1961, the commissioners noted, approximately 9.6 million Canadians were enrolled, in roughly equal proportion, in either insurance industry or prepayment plans. These plans covered medical and related bills but excluded hospital services covered under provincial hospital insurance plans. The insurance industry, now referring to its members as "multiple carriers," offered discount premium rates to those covered under group plans, while charging individual subscribers more. In group contracts, the report found, premium rates were on average 37 percent higher than the amount the companies paid out in benefits, the difference going to administration, taxes, and profits, collectively and mysteriously referred to as "overhead." For individual contracts, premiums ranged between 2 and 2.5 times the amount paid out in benefits to subscribers. In 1961, insurance companies received almost $85 million in group contract premiums and paid just over $63 million in benefits, while the corresponding figures for individuals approached $12.8 million and $5.7 million, respectively.

The prepayment plans "did not make quite the same distinction between 'insurable' and 'non-insurable'" people as the commercial plans did. However, they did impose age limitations and waiting periods "to guard against an adverse selection of risks" and competed with private insurers for group and nongroup contracts. Prepayment insurers earned over $109 million in group contract premiums while paying about $92 million in benefits, a margin of 18.5 percent. Individual subscribers paid more than $16 million in premiums, 11.4 percent above the $14 million they received in benefits. While operating on a nonprofit basis, the TCMP plans nonetheless were an important source of revenue for the medical profession.

Such statistics did not add a great deal of credibility to the arguments put forward by the medical profession and the industry for a subsidy approach, which even a casual observer could see would be a very expensive way to provide coverage for Canada's 7.5 million uninsured. But the premium and benefit comparisons were only part of the picture. The commissioners found that while prepayment plans paid on average only 80 percent of the cost of all physician services, commercial insurers paid only a third of such expenses for those covered by a group contract and between 21 and 45 percent of costs incurred by individuals. The difference between physician fees and insured reimbursements was made up by deductibles. "Such contracts," the commissioners noted dryly, "although providing a greater degree of protection, are still inadequate."

The CMA, TCMP, and insurance industry did not concern themselves with the whole spectrum of health care, nor did they advocate the privatization of hospital insurance. Instead, they doggedly argued for public subsidies to enable poor and poor-risk Canadians to subscribe to private plans for physician services. (Whereas the TCMP supported government subsidies to enable the uninsurable and low-income or poor to enroll in nonprofit physician-sponsored plans only, the insurance industry joined with the CMA to advocate subsidies for all insurers, whether nonprofit or for-profit.) The income ceilings they proposed were roughly equivalent to those established in the medical profession's own plans during the mid-1940s. For example, MSA-BC covered employees who earned less than $2400 a year in 1945. The ceilings proposed by the medical profession and the insurance industry in their submissions to the Hall Commission were $2000 for family heads with a rise of between $300 and $550 for each dependant. People earning above these thresholds would pay the full premiums charged by insurers. Using the industry's data, the CMA argued that approximately 3 million Canadians would require some assistance in obtaining medical insurance, all of whom, of course, would have to be means tested to verify their claims to eligibility. The insurance industry presumably would continue to means-test the health status of its subscribers.

If the insurance protection offered by private companies was inadequate, the calculations setting income ceilings for subsidies also left a lot to be desired in the eyes of the commissioners. The Royal Commission was concerned with the full spectrum of health care for Canadians, not just with physician services, and so this is where it began in evaluating the CMA-CHIA subsidy proposals. First, it calculated the full cost of premiums for medical, surgical, and hospital care, drugs, optical and dental services, and nursing care. These figures were then compared to data on Canadian incomes in 1961.

The commissioners calculated that the average family of four would have to spend $346 a year for health services in order to meet all of its health needs. "On the assumption that no one should pay more than 5 per cent [of his or her annual income], a single person earning $2,500 or more and a family head earning $6,900 or more would be able to meet his premium in full," the commissioners wrote. Almost 70 percent of individuals and over 84 percent of family heads in 1961 earned below this amount and therefore would be entitled to some level of subsidy if they passed a means test.

Using these figures, the commission estimated that between 54 and 75 percent of Canadians would qualify for subsidy assistance. The most optimistic estimate showed that between 9.9 and 14.1 million people, out of a population of some 18 million, would have had to submit themselves to a means test in 1961 to qualify for a government subsidy. Projected income and population increases showed that by 1971 between 40 and 60 percent of Canadians would require means testing to determine their eligibility. "This would pose a formidable task in terms of organizing administrative machinery, extra costs which Canadians cannot afford, and a method of examining the individual which, in the opinion of many Canadians, is contrary to the dignity of man."

The commission's rejection of the CMA-CHIA subsidy proposals was based on solid statistical and ethical grounds. But what of the "health services approach" advocated by that sweeping designation referred to as "consumer groups"? Like many others in this category, the Canadian Labour Congress (CLC) maintained that the Royal Commission should not be focussing on insurance at all, but rather on the question of whether health should be a public service, like education. The CLC said all Canadians should have access to health care by right of citizenship, and not on the basis of whether they obtained public insurance. The CLC estimated that between 90 and 95 percent of union members were covered under group health plans negotiated in their collective agreements with employers. However only 20 to 45 percent of health costs were met by private insurers – figures in line with the commission's own calculations – and the CLC believed 45 percent was "a very liberal upper estimate."

The trade union movement was sharply critical of the proposed public subsidy for private insurance and of any plan that would simply extend insurance coverage but maintain the status quo of private physician and health-care delivery. In its written brief, the CLC's position was unequivocal: "We favour a system of public health care that will be universal in application and comprehensive in coverage. We favour a system that will present no economic barrier between the service and those who need it. We are opposed to any provision which will require some people to submit themselves to a means test in order to obtain service. We look to a system of health care that will be regarded as a public service and not as an insurance mechanism."

Fee-for-service, or "piecework," was rejected by the CLC in favour of salaries for physicians. It saw a program that was free of direct charges at point-of-service and was administered through provincial departments of public health. The CLC, along with many other "consumer groups," also urged that broader objectives be included in any public health plan, including preventive services, drugs, dental services, home care, and financial provision for those disabled because of illness or injury. A progressive income tax policy, including an "upward revision in corporation tax," would enable Canadians to contribute to a national health program on a fair and equitable basis.

It is disappointing that the commissioners did not undertake a thorough analysis of the proposals from groups advocating a "health as public service" model. Their report included no cost estimates of such a proposal, nor did they contemplate a health-care system in which private provision of services would play no role whatsoever. They rejected England's National Health Service as a workable model for Canada (in large part because of its salary and capitation payment methods for doctors), yet noted in passing that Britons delivered 37 percent of medical services outside of hospital compared to only 2 percent in Canada's much more expensive hospital-based and physician-directed system. And while the British spent 3.25 percent of their Gross National Product (GNP) on a full public health program with little private-sector participation, well over half of Canada's 4.17 percent of GNP for health was financed by the government but delivered almost entirely by the private sector.[1]

A number of groups who supported the public service model were prepared to accept a national public health insurance program as a compromise. The United Church of Canada supported a public plan that, minimally, would be "universal (including all citizens within its provisions); comprehensive (including various medical and related needs in co-operation with the medical, nursing, dental, pharmaceutical and other related professions); and national (with the various provincial plans coordinated in a nation-wide program)." This closely resembled the type of health-care system recommended by the Royal Commission in its final report, but it was less than the vision articulated by a number of organizations that saw Canada's public education system as the appropriate model for the delivery and administration of medical services.

The commissioners flatly rejected a full public health-services program, referring to such an arrangement as "a system in which all providers of health services are functionaries under the control of the state," a description borrowed from the Canadian Medical Association. Instead they opted for a tax-supported public insurance model as the mechanism through which a self-regulated, privately administered health system would be financed, supplemented by federal grants where needed but "free of government control or domination." The public payment/private delivery approach recommended by the Royal Commission was, in many ways, the typical Canadian compromise, a halfway model between the for-profit, market-oriented approach so aggressively defended and promoted by the private insurance companies and the medical profession (with staunch backing from big business), and the tax-based public system urged by a broad number of people who used, or might use, health services.

The report's unifying theme and greatest strength was its call for a universal and comprehensive health insurance system characterized by "uniform terms and conditions" in every part of the country. "This is what Canada and the provinces working together should do," the commissioners stated. "It is not an idealist's dream, but a practical programme within Canada's ability, financially and practically," as had been amply demonstrated in Saskatchewan. Such a program would require full cooperation between Ottawa and the provinces, and a leadership role "which must be accepted by the Federal Government" to ensure that Canadians had access to the full spectrum of insured services to which they were entitled.

The injection of public funds into the health-care sector, the commissioners said, would not only remove barriers to access, but would also act as a powerful economic stimulant. The national unemployment rate in the early 1960s hovered at 7 percent, an unacceptably high figure that threatened the future of many thousands of young people. "Increasing manufacturing output has not been accompanied by corresponding increases in employment," the commissioners noted, because of technological change and the increased participation of foreign producers in the Canadian market. "It has been mainly the rising rates of production of government and other services sectors, along with the capital investment that this has required, which has prevented the level of unemployment rising to levels even higher than those actually recorded."

The commissioners argued that public expenditures giving all Canadians access to health services would stimulate the economy and create needed jobs. Government programs, they said, were needed to support economic growth, and economic growth made government programs possible: "The higher the level of per capita income, the higher the percentage of the national income devoted to public service tends to be. Fundamentally, the development of government is part and parcel of the whole process of economic growth."

In a refrain familiar to many Canadians in the 1990s, the Report of the Royal Commission noted that in 1961, expenditures by Canadians on all drugs "are equivalent to 95% of the outlay on physicians' services, with prescribed drugs representing about 43% of medical expenditures." The commissioners recommended the establishment of a National Drug Formulary and bulk purchasing by provincial governments to take advantage of available discounts, but said drug prices were so high that the cost of full coverage would be prohibitive. They recommended, instead, coverage under a Prescription Drug Benefit plan, cost-shared 50-50 with patients, but warned that "either the industry itself will make these drugs available at the lowest possible cost, or it will be necessary for [the] government to do so."

Interestingly, the Royal Commission urged that a plan to eliminate drug patents be delayed until 1969. Patents were seen by many policymakers in Ottawa as a restrictive trade practice because they gave large, mainly foreign, pharmaceutical companies a monopoly on drugs in Canada. In the end, the government decided not to remove patents, but it set the patent period at five years. In addition, the government implemented a system that allowed Canadian-based drug manufacturers to copy and market generic forms of patented medicines at lower prices, giving these young companies access to their home market. Less than thirty years later, Brian Mulroney's Conservative government would extend drug patents to an unprecedented twenty years and prohibit generic copying during the patent period – necessary steps, the prime minister explained, towards free and unrestricted trade.

To achieve the objectives of a full medicare program, the Royal Commission said that private spending on health should be replaced with public spending for all medical services. Such a plan should provide dental and optical services for children, expectant mothers, and welfare recipients, and include prescription drugs, prosthetics, and home care. Provinces would determine the timing for and the priorities in introducing each service under the medicare program. The commissioners estimated that by 1971, 85 percent of Canada's total spending on health would be financed publicly, compared to 55 percent in 1961 (a figure that included provincial hospital insurance plans and medical services for welfare recipients). On a per capita basis, public health expenditures (in constant 1961 dollars) would rise to $204 a year, while private expenditures would increase to $36 annually.

The commissioners grappled with the financing and constitutional requirements of such a large scheme. In the plan they put forward, governments would first establish adequate standards of services. Cost sharing between federal and provincial governments (a system known as "conditional grants-in-aid" because federal transfer payments were conditional on provincial compliance with national criteria) could "be used to create a structure of health services ... that is in keeping with Canada's federal structure while providing a high level of health care for all Canadians regardless of where they live." Second, provinces and territories would administer their own programs, but financing would be shared with the federal government.

This second requirement, however, raised the issue of provinces' unequal capacity to support national criteria. How could "uniform terms and conditions" be obtained when provincial capacity to pay even 50 percent of the costs was so unequal across the country, the commissioners asked. "The fact that resources, and economic conditions and progress are not uniform throughout Canada," meant that poorer provinces would be forced "to impose a tax burden above the national average" to meet national criteria. This was inherently unfair. The commissioners recommended that the federal and provincial governments share the costs for health spending equally. While acknowledging that poorer provinces would still face problems maintaining uniform terms and conditions even under this 50-50 shared cost formula, the commissioners declined to comment on "how far the present system [of shared cost arrangements] meets the needs of the federal government and the provinces" because such an evaluation was "beyond the terms of reference of this Commission."

After the Hall Commission

Responses to the Royal Commission's unanimous report in mid-1964 ranged from jubilation on the part of medicare proponents to bitter shock and disappointment on the part of the private insurance industry, big business, and the Canadian medical profession. Many doctors expressed legitimate concerns about potential interference from politicians who counted votes and measured public opinion when they made spending decisions – decisions between health and roads, for example, or between health and deficits. However, such decisions were also made by both the private insurance industry and the doctor-sponsored prepayment plans – decisions about what was "medically necessary," who was or was not insurable, and what was or was not appropriate treatment – and they considered this a paramount right. In the fight over medicare in Saskatchewan, and later during the federal government's deliberations on the same issue, the voices and concerns of doctors trying to balance their professional autonomy with a universal system of health care were drowned out by the rhetoric about socialism and free enterprise.

The CMA, in particular, ignored the principles that moved many physicians to fight for equitable access and fair compensation during the dark days of the Depression. Instead the association felt betrayed by the Royal Commission. The hope of the profession in urging such a commission in the first place had been to remove the medicare issue from "the hectic arena of political controversy," an arena in which 80 percent of Canadians continued to support national health insurance. The CMA-CHIA strategy had been to move the discussion away from the glare of public scrutiny, delay any federal action until the issue was a distant memory in the minds of the Canadian people, and thereby ensure a "socialistic" health program would never see the light of day. Clearly, this strategy had not worked.

The recommendations were now in the hands of a minority Liberal government led by Lester Pearson and made up of young, aggressive members of Parliament who were moving swiftly into leadership positions within the party. Many of these MPs, including Judy LaMarsh, Allan MacEachen, Walter Gordon, and Herb Gray, were strong supporters of a national health program, and medicare was also supported by the Liberal party's general membership. However, many other MPs were opposed, notably Mitchell Sharp who led the charge within the cabinet.

Then there was the New Democratic Party, which held the balance of power in Ottawa when the Hall Commission released its report and again after the national election in November 1965. There was no doubt in anyone's mind that the NDP would support the Hall report, and many thought it would vote against the government and force an election if the Liberals attempted to water down the recommendations. As well as playing an active and independent role led by Tommy Douglas and Stanley Knowles in the House of Commons, the NDP lent strategic support to Liberals urging implementation of the program recommended by the Royal Commission.

The first act of the government was to appoint fourteen committees under the Ministry of Health to study the Hall report and draft proposals on how its recommendations might be captured in legislation. These were submitted to another committee made up of senior officials from the Health and Finance ministries and the Privy Council. There were two issues that challenged the government at this stage: federal-provincial cost sharing; and how a national program in an area of provincial jurisdiction should – or could – be implemented.

The issue of shared cost programs was a sensitive one in the mid-1960s. Conditional grants-in-aid, as the programs were called, tied federal contributions to provincial compliance with national criteria. The provinces were moving defiantly against what they considered to be federal intrusion into "their" jurisdictions to ensure national criteria were being properly applied. Growing nationalist sentiment in Québec had reinforced that province's discomfort with Ottawa's use of federal cash payments to control the provincial agenda under the guise of shared cost programs. Québec recently had received corporate tax credits from Ottawa and had won the right to establish a public pension plan separate from the national plan then in place. In addition, many provinces opposed federal audits of provincial accounts and, like Québec, opposed the "tied aid" principle underlying shared cost programs. With provincial opposition to a national health program of any kind coming from Alberta, Ontario, and British Columbia, Ottawa was anxious to ensure its proposed funding formula and national standards would not be part of the controversy.

Just over a year after the Hall report's release, a federal-provincial conference was convened to discuss "ways in which federal and provincial action can most effectively contribute to programs that will provide health services to Canadians on a comprehensive basis." Prime Minister Pearson outlined the main elements of a national medicare plan that would be based on an "understanding" between the federal and provincial governments rather than on "detailed agreements." Instead of "criteria," the medicare plan would embrace national "principles": comprehensive coverage of physician services, universality, publicly administered health insurance, and the portability of benefits, meaning residents would still be eligible for care when they were absent from their home province or when they moved to another province.

Pearson reassured the provinces that medicare would not adopt the conditional grants-in-aid model for federal transfer payments. Rather, once the provinces embraced national principles, Ottawa would detach itself from the administrative and budgetary details involved in administering the program. The federal transfer would total 50 percent of average national per capita costs so that provinces with lower per capita incomes would nonetheless be entitled to the same amount as wealthier provinces. So, for example, if the national cost per person was $300, each province would be entitled to $150 for each resident. Poorer provinces with lower per capita incomes would receive enough federal money to bring them up to the national average health expenditure per person. Ottawa would finance its portion of the cost from new tax revenues, an option available to the provinces as well.

As Ottawa fiddled with funding formulas, the CMA, the private insurance industry, and their provincial allies in Alberta, Ontario, and British Columbia were organizing against medicare. For the provinces opposed to a national program, public administration and universality might mean (and in the case of Alberta definitely would mean) either a substantial redesign of existing policies to bring them in line with national principles or the loss of federal transfer payments. For both the CMA and the CHIA, the adoption of these principles would spell the end of private insurance in the health-care field, the end of extra billing, and the end of a lucrative source of profits.

When Bill C-227, the Medical Care Insurance Act, was tabled in the House of Commons on July 12, 1966, it was obvious that the federal government had got the message, not from the Canadian people, but from the medical profession and the insurance industry. The legislation captured the four principles enunciated by the prime minister a year earlier, plus several new details. Most important among these was a redefinition of the term "publicly administered," which now allowed provincial governments to contract private insurers to provide coverage on a nonprofit basis, and a clause allowing doctors to opt out and directly bill their patients. The principle of universality – at least in theory – would be protected in provincial health plans. Patients would be reimbursed for the publicly insured portion of the services they obtained.

Despite these compromises, the CMA-CHIA alliance continued to attack the plan, especially the principle of universality – what the CMA-CHIA referred to as a system based on "compulsion." Under Ottawa's proposed medicare scheme, the alliance warned, Canadians would no longer have the freedom to choose whether or not they would be insured or who would insure them, a freedom viewed by the alliance as a fundamental tenet of any free-enterprise, democratic society. A patient's freedom to make "private arrangements" with his or her own doctor would be seriously impaired, charged the alliance, and instead of having over 120 private insurers to choose from, Canadians would be forced to insure under a single government "monopoly."

A public opinion poll conducted in September 1965 indicated that these arguments were having the desired effect. But the wording of the poll conducted by the Canadian Institute of Public Opinion was hardly neutral. "Do you think the medicare program should be a compulsory one, in which every Canadian would have to join," the questionnaire asked, "or do you think it should be a voluntary [i.e., private] plan, in which Canadians themselves could decide whether or not to join?" While most Canadians supported a medicare program, not surprisingly 52 percent said they favoured a "voluntary" plan in which they could be free to choose whether or not to participate, rather than a "compulsory" approach.

If confusion reigned in the public opinion polls, the divisions within the Liberal cabinet were threatening to scuttle the implementation of medicare altogether. The government's original target date for implementation was the occasion of Canada's centenary, July 1, 1967. Many leading Liberals were anxious to proceed, both because the day was a highly symbolic one and would bring maximum public exposure to the momentous event and because further delays could lead to further compromises. This was an important consideration given that the CMA and the insurance companies had a powerful ally in the cabinet – Finance Minister Mitchell Sharp.

The business community, the insurance industry, and the CMA also had a powerful new economic weapon to use against such a costly proposition as medicare promised to be. With the federal deficit projected to increase substantially in the latter part of the 1960s, and inflation applying upward pressure, businessmen and the country's main media outlets questioned the wisdom of introducing medicare in an "overheated" economy. Thus prompted, Sharp began mobilizing his cabinet colleagues to support a postponement of medicare's launch to July 1968, giving the economy time to cool down. Pearson was still committed to a centennial year start date, but while he was out of the country, Sharp, in his capacity as deputy prime minister, unexpectedly announced in the House of Commons that the date had been postponed to the following year. A furor ensued, with Health Minister Allan MacEachen threatening to resign from cabinet and Walter Gordon and Judy LaMarsh publicly attacking Sharp, the private insurance industry, and the medical profession – the "opponents of medicare." In subsequent and heated cabinet discussions it was agreed that July 1968 would be the launch date, and Pearson made a commitment that there would be no further delays.

The landmark Medical Care Insurance Act passed in the House of Commons with only two dissenting votes on December 8, 1966. Implemented on July 1, 1968, the bill was seen by many Canadians as a first step – a significant step to be sure, but one taken on the way to a more encompassing system of public health-care delivery. For insurers, the enactment of medicare legislation was a serious setback, but not a final defeat. For these interests the introduction of universal public health insurance brought about a major reorganization but not a cessation of their operations.

FOUR

Medicare: Thirty Years Down the Road

The implementation of medicare varied from province to province, but great efforts were made across the country to minimize the impact on the insurance industry and the medical profession. Most provinces moved within a couple of years to merge their existing hospital insurance programs into new plans that covered a comprehensive range of physician and hospital services. Some provinces charged a nominal premium to supplement the tax revenues they allocated to health insurance.

Provincial variations

Under the federal Act, provincial governments could establish a public authority that could, in turn, designate a public or private agency to administer the health plan, and many chose this option. British Columbia, for example, originally designated MSA-BC, the private, physician-sponsored plan, as an "approved carrier." The insurer simultaneously reorganized its extended health coverage to include services not on the province's health insurance plan. Manitoba established a Crown corporation that took over physician-run Manitoba Medical Services. Nova Scotia arranged the administration of its health plan through Maritime Medical Care, the physician-sponsored plan, while Prince Edward Island, New Brunswick, and Newfoundland administered their medicare plans directly. Saskatchewan, of course, had already established its plan by the time Ottawa enacted the national health program, and the province continued to administer its insurance system without outside agencies.

Governments in three provinces enacted legislation that broke the pattern established in other jurisdictions. Ernest Manning's Social Credit government in Alberta had opposed medicare from the outset and was reluctant to exclude the powerful insurance industry from the health-care field. The province rejected participation in Ottawa's national program in April 1967 when it set up the Alberta Health Plan. Under the plan, the health minister was given the authority to appoint approved insurance companies and to negotiate a fee with each insurer for the administration of the plan. This was essentially the same program the province had established in conjunction with private insurers and the medical association in 1963. But mounting public criticism of Alberta's refusal to support Ottawa's national criteria and thereby qualify for federal funding forced the province to bring its medicare scheme in line with the national program. In 1969 a provincial commission was established to administer the plan, and both commercial and nonprofit insurers were excluded.

Ontario, another vociferous opponent of Ottawa's Medical Care Insurance Act, decided initially against participating in the national scheme. However, with other provinces jumping on board and with strong public support for Ottawa's medicare program, the Conservative government of Premier John Robarts initiated discussions with commercial and nonprofit insurers to establish a consortium to administer a provincial health plan. The physician-sponsored plan decided to turn over its operation to the government, but twenty-nine commercial insurers agreed to act as sub-agents of the consortium on a no-profit, no-loss basis. Agreements were reached between the insurance companies and HealthCo, acting as an agent of the provincial government. Under the agreement, the twenty-nine commercial insurers administered medical coverage for some 2.5 million Ontarians for a 5 percent fee, while 4 million residents were covered by the government-run Ontario Health Insurance Plan (OHIP). This arrangement – which demonstrated that a "government monopoly" was more efficient and less costly than a platoon of private insurers – lasted for two and a half years, at which time the province amalgamated its hospital and medical services plans and brought the administration of health insurance under a single public roof.[1]

Québec's health plan went into effect on November 1, 1970, and was unique in Canada for a number of reasons. Unlike the other provinces, Québec embarked on a plan to provide health services as part of a broad social benefits system that included a comprehensive range of public services, from medical care to social assistance. Quebeckers would have to be included on the province's insurance plan to obtain health and physician services, but these would be delivered mainly in the public sector. This differed from the rest of the country, which did not view health as a social service, but rather as a publicly financed private enterprise. Québec, unlike the other provinces, also rejected public payment to physicians who opted out of the public plan. Instead, the Québec government's medicare legislation included a goal to replace doctors' fee-for-service payments with salaries or capitation fees. This direction was assisted by the establishment of local community service centres in the 1980s.

The Québec government envisioned a system of "total" care, delivered in local and community-based health centres staffed by a team of medical and paramedical professionals. This attempt to "gradually abandon the traditional closed (medical) model and adopt a more open social model" integrated preventive and curative programs, while maintaining hospitals as acute-care providers. Hospitals and most health services were placed directly in the public sector. Finally, the government put in place a system of comprehensive and continuous care, including dental and outpatient services, publicly administered and under local control through twelve regional councils. The Québec health plan split physicians along historical lines, with general practitioners who accepted or supported the plan on one side, and specialists, who did not, on the other. Specialists initiated strike action in

1970 in an unsuccessful attempt to force the government to withdraw the health plan's enabling legislation. But while specialists failed in their efforts, the deficit hysteria of the late 1980s and 1990s proved a more effective weapon against Québec's innovative system of health-care financing and delivery. As in the rest of Canada, the province reacted to federal cuts in transfer payments by closing hospitals and delisting services.[2]

In December 1969 the TCMP surrendered its national charter, but its twelve provincial organizations had varying degrees of success in the new world of public health insurance. Between 1968 and 1969 the number of people covered by nonprofit insurers dropped from 8 million to 2 million, a decline that, not surprisingly, put many plans out of business. With their Blue Cross counterparts, physician-sponsored plans became the nonprofit alternatives to commercial carriers for insured health benefits not included on public plans. Those that were able to negotiate arrangements with provincial governments to administer public health insurance, or that managed to compete with the growing and increasingly aggressive commercial insurance industry, survived. Investor-owned companies, on the other hand, entered a period of restructuring and reorientation towards foreign markets, particularly those in the United States.[3]

By 1971 all provinces in Canada had established a system of public health insurance. In establishing their medicare programs, the provinces had chosen not to rigidly define what was and was not an insurable health-care service. Since most services were delivered either in a hospital, a mental health facility, or a doctor's office, the need for definitions was not an urgent one. There were grey areas – especially in the case of outpatient health services – but these had been addressed by the Royal Commission, which had recommended, for example, that physiotherapy services be included on provincial insurance plans. But inpatient physiotherapy was defined as a hospital service. What if these services were delivered by a professional in private practice outside the hospital sector? There were no national answers or definitions for questions like this, and the provinces were, by and large, left to decide for themselves.

To qualify for federal funds, provinces were required to publicly administer an insurance program covering hospital and physician services on a nonprofit basis – that is, the insurance had to be publicly administered and nonprofit, but the services could be delivered in the private and for-profit sector. Under the medicare program, hospitals and physicians were prevented from delivering publicly insured services and charging patients an extra amount above what they received from the province. Except in Québec, where hospitals were in the public sector, acute-care facilities operate on a nonprofit basis administering publicly insured hospital services. However, there was nothing to prevent them from supplying and charging market rates for services not on the public insurance plan.

EPF and the death of a thousand cuts

Few Canadians could understand the intricacies of the health-care system and the complicated legal framework and funding relationships that were set in place. The details are still largely unknown to this day. But what was understood, and deeply valued, was the independence Canadians gained in the new health system. The ability to prevent illness from becoming a catastrophe or a tragedy, the right to see a doctor for a medical check-up or a broken leg, the assurance that one's children would not be felled by a treatable injury were all benefits of medicare. Many people who supported medicare during the long years of heated debates preceding its introduction had to endure the humiliation of risk assessments, means tests, and rejection – not to mention the suffering and pain associated with untreated disease and sickness. But their offspring, coming of age in the early 1970s, would never experience the fear of even mild illnesses that was common among their parents. It was now up to a new generation to protect and improve what had been bequeathed. As Canadians' experiences with health care diverged more and more sharply from those of their neighbours to the south, and as medicare proved its worth on a day-by-day, person-by-person basis, the dismantling of what became known as Canada's "most cherished social program" became a perilous undertaking for governments at every level.

Nonetheless, under continued political pressure from medicare's opponents, governments began to contain and then erode Canada's publicly funded and largely nonprofit health-care system. While cost containment may be a laudable goal, it has usually been accompanied by measures that weaken public authority and expand the role of for-profit companies in health care. Six years after medicare was established coast to coast, Ottawa – embarked on an anti-inflation crusade – targeted its funding relationship with the provinces in an attempt to rein in federal spending on social programs and health care.

In 1977 the Liberals passed the Established Programs Financing Act (EPF), which changed the 50-50 cost-sharing formula used to fund health care. The legislation also ended federal responsibility to contribute a fixed percentage to provincial health spending, signalling a decreased role for Ottawa in health-care matters. Under EPF the federal government put in place a more complex system of transfer payments, grants, and tax points that all spelled less money to the provinces over the long run. Provincial governments were given the power to set funding levels for health services without federal interference. The immediate result was a relatively modest drop in federal cash transfers, reductions that would assume mammoth proportions in the coming years.[4]

More importantly, while EPF cash transfers met provincial demands for unconditional grants, they weakened the ability of the federal government to enforce national standards in two ways. Through the EPF program Ottawa significantly and legislatively weakened its role in and control over matters affecting health-care policy. Second, EPF reduced Ottawa's financial support to the provinces, support that was vital to the economic and structural stability in the sector. Under EPF, Ottawa was able to introduce further reductions in cash transfers for health through a budgetary process instead of a public policy approach that required lengthy, not to mention public, negotiations with the provinces. Despite the federal government's reassurances that it too saw medicare as a cherished program, the move sparked protests led by unions and public-health-care advocates. Activists formed the Canadian Health Coalition to fight further attacks on the health system, drawing inspiration from the earlier struggles to establish medicare. The coalition remains active – and growing – in the 1990s.

The biggest challenge it confronts is the fact that few Canadians understand how the funding system works – or can work. And because the changes during the last two decades have been so complex and arcane, it has been hard to generate an organized and broad-based outcry against them. From the perspective of many politicians, the less Canadians know about how the health-care system works, the better.

In the early 1980s, many doctors, despite the steep increases in income they had experienced under medicare, began complaining that the fee schedules they negotiated with ministries of health compared poorly to the income levels their U.S. colleagues enjoyed (a claim that was true if one ignored the fact that U.S. doctors paid an average of $30,000 a year for liability insurance). Under the Medical Care Insurance Act, doctors had retained the right to opt out of medicare and charge whatever they – and private insurers who paid patients' bills – liked. But doctors were not prepared to abandon a system that treated them as independent entrepreneurs on the one hand, and guaranteed them a high enough level of income to offset the administrative and other costs of running a business on the other. Simply put, many physicians wanted to make more money than provincial governments were willing or able to give them under medicare. They wanted to reap the rewards of public payments for physician services and also extra-bill patients to increase their incomes. If they were not allowed to do this, they threatened a mass exodus of doctors to the south. These physicians aroused more hostility than sympathy among the public, who demanded that extra billing and opting out be unequivocally abolished.

And they were. In 1984 the Canada Health Act was passed unanimously in the House of Commons. Not only did it abolish extra billing, it also strengthened the principles underlying the health-care system and Ottawa's role in maintaining national standards. While most Canadians believe the Act encompassed the full spectrum of health-care services, in fact the legislation set out and defined, loosely, five criteria that would govern the operation of provincial health insurance plans and that must be met "before payment may be made under the [EPF] Act of 1977." The legislation went further than its 1966 predecessor, raising the "principles" of medicare to the level of criteria and enabling Ottawa to withhold its cash transfers if the provinces failed to comply with the rules of the Act. The five criteria were:

1. Provincial health insurance plans had to be publicly administered and nonprofit. Hospitals and physicians could not charge patients for services insured on the provincial plan. However, they could charge for health services not included on the public health plan. And the Act did not apply to Canada's extensive employer-funded workers' compensation system, which paid for services required by workers because of a workplace injury or illness.

2. Plans had to "insure all insured health services." The lack of definitions in the Act regarding the nature of an insured service created a new line of business for the consulting industry in Canada. Along with hospitals and health corporations, consultants have tried to define the term "medically necessary services," which was inserted but not explained in the legislation. The term has been at the centre of debates about what is and what is not insurable. For example, dental services were included in the 1984 criteria, as well as, "where permitted, services rendered by other health practitioners," for example, rehabilitation services delivered by a physiotherapist in private practice. Few provinces have ever covered dental care, while coverage for physiotherapy delivered in private practice is uneven across the country.

3. Everyone who was on a provincial health plan had to have access to insured services on equal terms and conditions. Simply, what one person got, all were entitled to. This principle of universality made it illegal to discriminate against a person on the basis of pre-existing conditions, age, gender, income, or any other characteristic. This clause alone effectively removed the private insurance industry from the provision of medically necessary health care, since it was unwilling to drop its degrading risk assessment policies, a move that would have had a negative impact on profits.

4. Insurance coverage had to be portable for up to three months and available to people temporarily out of their home province or out of the country. This meant that those establishing residency in another province received continuous coverage and that those vacationing outside the country were protected. The portability provisions of the Act with respect to out-of-country coverage have been seriously eroded.

5. Provincial health plans, in the language of the Act, had to provide "reasonable access by insured persons to insured health services unprecluded or unimpeded, either directly or indirectly, by charges or other means." This banned extra billing and allowed Ottawa to withhold transfer payments to provinces that turned a blind eye to the practice. Ottawa argued, correctly, that it needed a monetary tool to bring about compliance, but federal politicians were also recasting the objective of federal funding from one that would establish equity among the provinces to one that would be used to whip them into line. This fifth guideline also required that doctors and dentists be paid a "reasonable compensation" and that hospitals receive payments for "the cost of insured health services." If hospitals had been designated as public institutions, they would have received all their funding from provincial governments, not just a reimbursement for the costs of delivering publicly insured care.[5]

The Canada Health Act provided Ottawa with an effective "no compliance, no cash" lever with which to enforce national standards. It served to strengthen not only the legal framework within which the health sector functions, but also the fight to defend longstanding principles held by the Canadian people. It weakened the 1980s push for free-market medicine and required doctors who wanted to bill patients over and above the fees negotiated with provincial governments to leave the public health plan, something that very few chose to do. The overriding belief among Canadians that everyone should have equal access to medical services regardless of ability to pay – a belief based on what health economist Robert Evans has described as a "deep-rooted suspicion of class-based systems of any kind" – was strongly reflected in the Act. And finally, the legislation provided Canadians with a protective barrier against aggressive corporate strategies that aimed to open up the health-care sector to private investment and profit making.

'No cash, no compliance'

Although the Canada Health Act received wide popular support across the country, the governing Liberals and their anti-inflation crusade did not. The election of the Progressive Conservatives under the leadership of Brian Mulroney in 1984 proved to be a disaster for the country's health-care system, bringing a series of cuts in EPF transfer payments to the provinces for health and post-secondary education in 1985, 1990, and 1991. The cumulative loss of revenue to provincial coffers during the Mulroney years amounted to $30 billion for health care alone, with another $6.5 billion drawn out of the system by the Chrétien Liberals. These were cuts that all provinces were reluctant, and most were unable, to offset.

The reductions in cash transfers also reduced the clout Ottawa was able to exert over provinces that failed to comply with the principles of the Canada Health Act. "No cash, no compliance" was the predictable response from many provincial capitals. It is hard to imagine that the Mulroney government did not anticipate this response, but it would not be of much concern to a government anxious to demonstrate that Canada could meet the new "global economy's" demands for reduced public-sector involvement in areas that promised lucrative investment opportunities. Caught between Ottawa's withdrawal of federal funds and lack of a national vision for health on the one hand, and their own constitutional claims to jurisdiction over health care on the other, most provinces maintained an ominous silence, choosing instead to close hospitals, delist services, and ponder the meaning of "medically necessary."[6]

Provincial funding cutbacks or inadequate funding increases to hospitals and other service providers (excluding doctors) mirrored the cuts in federal transfer payments. There was, at the same time, a parallel redistribution of public and private health expenditures. In 1975 the public funded more than three quarters (76.4 percent) of the total health-care bill, while private insurance arrangements or direct out-of-pocket payments covered 23.6 percent. By 1986 the split was 73.3 percent public and 26.7 percent private, and in 1997 about 68 percent public and 32 percent private.

The oft-heard complaint expressed by critics of medicare (such as the *Globe and Mail* newspaper) that "Canada administers the most expensive public health-care program in the world" was and is untrue. According to the Organization for Economic Cooperation and

Development (OECD), in 1993 the country ranked sixteenth among the twenty-four leading industrial nations when public spending was calculated as part of the total health picture. But when overall health expenditures – which combined both public and private spending – were calculated, Canada placed second – a position that in 1995 dropped to fifth place behind the United States, Germany, France, and Switzerland. That drop was entirely the result of public spending cuts. While private spending held steady between 1992 and 1994, public spending fell from 7.5 percent of GDP to 6.9 percent.[7]

Public fears escalated about the future of medicare, stoked by media reports that the program had "added substantially to Canada's staggering debt" and was "lumbering toward disintegration." These claims were exacerbated by politicians, most of whom continued to implement funding cuts while avoiding public debate about whether such actions were necessary. The absence of definitions in the Canada Health Act allowed provinces to argue on the grounds of "medical necessity," or unnecessity, when they decided to remove a service like annual physical or eye exams from public health plans. Once the service was removed, it could be covered by private insurers. Needless to say, the private insurance industry saw increased profits in the delisting activities of provincial governments.

But some federal bureaucrats argued that definitions of medical necessity would tie the hands of policymakers. What would have happened, they asked, if such definitions had been legislated in the mid-seventies when medical science seemed to come up with new discoveries on a daily basis? New treatments for new diseases such as AIDS would not have been included in the definition and therefore would not have been covered. The absence of definitions gave policymakers flexibility in deciding what would be covered under public health plans. This was an important feature for advocates of increased coverage both inside and outside of government. It could be argued, as well, that the ambiguity in the Canada Health Act was a blessing in disguise, giving federal policymakers, who often took the broader view and could be more reliable medicare supporters than their provincial counterparts, the ability to interpret the meaning of medical necessity more liberally.[8]

In all of these discussions about medical necessity, there was no debate at all about the private insurance industry, which presumably was charging higher and higher premiums for "unnecessary" medical services. In fact, much of the growing debate in business and media circles about the need for a definition of a medically necessary service in the Canada Health Act was initiated by private insurers. They, of course, wanted services to be delisted and were willing to offer advice on the difficult choices confronting policymakers.

The need for definitions was not felt by public policymakers when medicare was being set up, mainly because they, and Canadians generally, held many justifiable assumptions about health care. The first was that all health services were necessary – and therefore should be available without the barriers the market imposed. This made the question of medical necessity moot. The second assumption, and one that flowed from the first, was that individuals, groups, institutions, or entities involved in the delivery of health care – collectively known as providers – should operate on a nonprofit basis.

Thirty years on, many of the market principles espoused by corporate executives and investors permeate Canada's nonprofit health-care sector. Those who defend health-care profits believe that competition between providers is necessary to increase efficiency, eliminate waste, and lower costs. At the very least, they argue that productivity must be improved, especially in the hospital sector, and the management techniques – such as mass layoffs – that increased profits in factories and industrial plants should be employed in hospitals.

After thirty years of medicare, Canada's universal health-care system has maintained high levels of support. Across geographic, age, gender, racial, and class boundaries, Canadians know that committed leadership and financial support from the federal government is crucial to protect medicare. In a 1995 public survey by Ottawa-based Ekos Research Associates, nearly 80 percent of those polled said they wanted the federal government to either maintain or increase its role in the health-care sector, while 89 percent said Ottawa and the provinces should work together to improve the health-care system. In the same survey, only 6 percent of those polled said they preferred that private business be given responsibility for health care, compared to 71 percent who wanted governments to retain that role. In another survey by the same company, 84 percent rated equal access to health care for all Canadians and the quality of health-care services as the most important aspects of the system, while 60 percent rejected "queue jumping" by individuals able to pay for services.

Despite the ceaseless denigration of publicly supported health care by advocates of market competition and profits, Canadians have displayed a remarkable tenacity in their embrace of the system. Insurance and health industry officials also have been careful to declare their support for and commitment to Canadian values. But during the 1980s and 1990s, this support was laced with economic and pseudo-scientific analyses about the problems in health-care financing and delivery. Health care, said a growing chorus in the business community, was "in critical condition," raising the question of "whether Canada should consider reintroducing private enterprise to its medical system." In one way or another, the corporate sector was determined that Canadian health care was going to be reformed.[9]

FIVE

Recreating Health Care

The introduction of medicare in 1966 did not exclude private entities from delivering health-care services or, for that matter, from insuring them. On the contrary, the principles of public payment and private delivery of services were firmly embraced by the Hall Commission and in subsequent legislation. The Canada Health Act had incorporated the term "medically necessary" in its criteria in 1984, a caveat that enabled private insurers to develop and then expand a market niche in supplementary health benefits. The fears that Canada's insurance industry would be doomed with the advent of public health insurance proved to be not only inaccurate, but wildly off-base.

The expansion of public health insurance to cover both hospital and medical services in Canada pushed health insurers to restructure the domestic insurance industry and create a new market for insured health products and nonhospital, nonphysician services. The United States, too, was embarked on a major policy initiative that saw the introduction of a public health insurance program for the elderly, the disabled and the poor. While U.S. Medicare was much more modest than Canada's universal health-care program, it nonetheless cut into a lucrative market dominated by U.S. insurers. Thus, the reorganization of the industry was not unique to Canada, but rather was occurring throughout North America.

By the mid-1970s there were three groups that predominated in the health insurance business in Canada. The first group was made up of the old physician- and hospital-sponsored plans, which continued as nonprofit alternatives to the commercial insurance industry. The second group was composed of nonprofit insurers founded by progressive-minded and membership-based groups to provide extended health services to their members, for example, churches, trade unions and farmers' organizations. The third group was the commercial insurance industry that like its physician-sponsored counterparts had experienced a drop in the number of subscribers when medicare was introduced. However, unlike most of their nonprofit competitors, few insurance companies in Canada depended exclusively on premium income from the sale of accident and sickness policies. These insurers survived the curtailment of their activities in the health sector, becoming the main providers of supplementary health and life insurance policies to large employers. These companies also introduced an endless line of new products, such as kidnap and ransom insurance for corporate executives doing business in the uncertain political climates of countries around the globe.

By the end of the 1960s commercial insurers offered two classes of insurance in Canada. Life insurance included supplementary health (also known as extended health) benefits, annuities, and pension fund management, while general insurance covered liability, property and casualty, auto, and cargo. The two classes of insurance "products," as these intangible offerings were called, were sold by two predominant types of insurance companies: mutuals, "owned" – at least in principle – by the policyholders; and stock companies, owned – in fact – by shareholders.

The restructuring among commercial insurers was accompanied by a stunning increase in premium costs for products such as life and home insurance. This rise helped ease the loss of revenues that followed the introduction of medicare. Between 1961 and 1975 the cost of life insurance policies in Canada rose more than 48 percent, while home insurance increased by a whopping 421 percent. Despite the loss of much of the lucrative health insurance market, growth in the life insurance industry averaged 5.8 percent in each year from 1961 to 1985, compared to 4.1 percent a year in manufacturing over the same period. As the companies grew, so too did their financial assets, rising from $9.8 billion in 1961 to $19 billion ten years later.

The exposure of health insurance profits during the 1960s did little to alter the pattern of high premiums and low benefit payouts in the subsequent decades. In the mid-1980s, Helen Anderson, a former official with the Consumers' Association of Canada, echoed the complaints sounded two decades earlier when she said, "Life insurance claims each year are half of what [the companies] take in in premiums. Now if you always took in twice as much money as you paid out every year you can imagine how wealthy you'd be."

Wealthy, indeed. Today there are over 140 life and health insurance companies operating in Canada, employing more than 65,000 people. Worldwide premium income in 1995 exceeded $45 billion for the year, in addition to assets worth over $165 billion. But the assets and profits of the insurance industry are not distributed evenly among companies in this fiercely competitive sector. Four companies control nearly half the life insurance business, and the top ten companies rake in 75 percent of total direct premiums, while 84 percent control less than 1 percent of market share.

The growing private health dollar

The limits placed on health insurers when universal medicare was introduced were short lived. Spending on health in Canada is divided between "public" and "private" sources – that is, the public portion of each health dollar comes from individual and corporate taxes, while the rest is spent directly by individuals for private insurance and for uninsured products or services. (In 1997, combined public and private spending on health was $76 billion.)

This distinction is misleading, however, as nearly all spending comes from the pockets of individual income-earners. The public portion of health-care costs, derived from tax revenues, is used to fund insured services provided by doctors and hospitals. Public funds pay for the construction of hospitals and other facilities at the federal, provincial, territorial, and municipal levels. Taxes also fund public drug and mental health programs; pensions for people with disabilities; and health, dental, and optical services for aboriginal people, the elderly, children, and those on social assistance.

Although employers claim that the private portion of health-care expenditures is paid directly by them in the form of insurance premiums for supplementary health and dental benefits covering their employees, these costs are calculated as part of the total payroll package earned by employees. Thus it is income-earners who now pay nearly 30 percent of their "health dollar" to employers to obtain health insurance from private insurers, who in turn pay for services covered on supplementary benefits plans. In addition, employees often must pay an extra share of the insurance premium in the form of a co-payment, as well as deductibles on their purchases of services and products. When Canada's corporate elite complain that Canadians have a sense of entitlement, they are right: Canadians do claim entitlement to health care, and so they should, if for no other reason than almost every health-care dollar flows from their hands.

When governments reduce public funding for health care, the amount spent by employers on the benefits side of the wage package increases as insurers raise premiums to cover increasing costs and services delisted from public health plans. The response of employers trying to keep wages and benefits down is to pass these costs on to their employees in the form of higher co-payments to offset higher insurance premiums. Individual, or private, expenditures for health go up, government expenditures go down, and control shifts increasingly from elected officials responsible for the public pool of health dollars to employers who manage the pool in the private sector.

During the 1970s and most of the 1980s, private expenditures hovered between 23 percent and 25 percent of the total spent on health care. After 1988, private expenditures began to climb steadily as Ottawa embarked on massive cuts in the amount of money it transferred to the provinces for health – cuts that would total $36.5 billion by the end of the 1990s.[3] About one third of total health expenditures now flow through the insurance industry and consequently the portion of premium income derived from the sale of health policies has grown, too. While federal cuts in transfer payments to the provinces for health provide a backdrop to the rising profits earned in the health insurance market, there are several other factors that must be taken into account as well.

The first, and perhaps most important, is the removal, or delisting, of medical services from public health plans and the increased deductibles for prescription drugs. Delisting and deductibles increased as provincial governments passed on the costs of federal funding cuts to Canadians during the 1990s. The delisting of services from provincial plans threatens to turn Canada's public, comprehensive medicare system into a program of insurance for catastrophic illness, disease, and injury.

This was, in fact, the vision put forward in 1995 by Jean Chretien. Attempting to justify another $2.5 billion cut in federal health spending, Canada's prime minister said that medicare never was meant to cover "frills" such as eyeglasses, dental care, or emergency ambulance services. "Nobody loses his home because somebody has a problem with his teeth or his eyes," he said, apparently unaware that medicare has never included such items in spite of the intentions and requirements of the Canada Health Act. "If you have major surgery," he told Peter Gzowski, host of CBC's *Morningside*, "medicare was intended for that." Canada, Chretien said, should get back to its roots, when insurance protected sick people from bankruptcy. Canadians, he added, would have to accept a "no-frills" public medicare system from now on. Grant Hill, health critic for the Reform Party, was relieved. "This is the first crack," he said, "the first indication that they [the Liberals] realize really deep down what has to happen."[4]

The private health-insurance business is also expanding because governments are failing to insure many new services and procedures that can increase the independence and mobility of patients. Those who live with chronic conditions, for example, often struggle on a daily basis to maintain independence and control over their lives. The availability of home infusion equipment for hemophiliacs, or insulin pump therapy for diabetics, for example, can both improve the quality of life for many patients with these diseases and save the health-care system millions of dollars by precluding the need for expensive hospital or emergency treatment. Nonetheless, these new medical devices are not deemed medically necessary by provincial governments, so low- and middle-income Canadians who can afford neither the equipment nor the insurance premiums that might cover such purchases must do without.

While many patients need services they are not getting, many others are getting services they don't need. The corporate health sector has created markets for an array of health services and products that are unnecessary – and sometimes harmful – and from which they derive a sizeable part of their profits. Nowhere is this better illustrated than in the "OTC" – or over-the-counter – drug industry.

Global drug companies have exerted a great deal of effort and time to develop the over-the-counter drug market around the world. One OTC trade magazine, in an analysis of the Czech Republic – "tipped as one of the best OTC investment prospects among the countries of the former Eastern Bloc"- concluded in the mid-1990s that there was a "fundamental cultural barrier" to Western brand-name drugs for indigestion. When they experience gastrointestinal problems, complained the author, "[Czech] consumers choose to adjust their eating habits, rather than resorting to medication." Multinational drug sellers launched expensive and effective targeted advertising campaigns – called "adspends" – to overcome the problem and to convince Czechs that they could continue eating as usual if they took Western brands of medication. Drug multinationals also confronted another type of "barrier to market penetration" – high prices – but these were barriers the companies could live with.[5]

Such strategies have built an industry in North America and around the world for an array of health goods and services, many of which are medically unnecessary responses to problems that could be addressed through a change in diet, clean drinking water, education, higher incomes, better housing, less pollution, and an improved quality of life. The insurance industry has been a stalwart supporter of corporations that hawk a variety of questionable health products and services, jumping to include them in health insurance policies in spite of their dubious worth to patients. That's because the worth of health care as a commodity is assessed solely on the basis of profit and loss ratios, rather than on the basis of value. Needless to say, these health products have never been subjected to the same assessment of medical necessity that Canada's entire public health insurance system has undergone in recent years.

The global insurance industry

Czechoslovakia is not the only country in which health-care corporations confront cultural barriers. After Ottawa's $2.5 billion cut to medicare in early 1995, health-care entrepreneurs interested in stepping into the breach acknowledged they would have to "leap a cultural barrier" because "many Canadians oppose the idea of anyone making a profit from health care." The cultural challenge, the proponents of private sector medicine acknowledged, was monumental.

First, Canadians had to be convinced that governments were putting "excess money in the system." The insurance industry claimed that as much as 40 percent of public expenditures could be defined as excessive, and it argued that Canadians had to accept decreased government spending in the public interest. Second, insurers had to show that while public spending was excessive, private spending was not – was, in fact, necessary. As George Ward, head of Canada's provincial Blue Cross insurers put it, "If [governments] are going to take all this money out of health care, they've got to allow people vehicles to self-protect" against illnesses no longer adequately addressed by medicare. Third, the insurance industry had to convince Canadians to abandon their stubborn notions about "entitlement" and accept that access to health care was not a fundamental right, but rather a question of money – and those willing to spend the most should get the access to the best.[6]

From the perspective of many in the corporate community, the so-called "entitlement mentality" among Canadians was undermining efforts to deal effectively with the problems besetting the economy, in particular the deficit. Corporations reasoned that government spending on health should be cut back so that individuals who wish to spend can do so on their own, rather than adding to the deficit burden future generations have to carry. Deficit reduction during the 1980s was a priority for the corporate sector, including banks and insurance companies. In June 1993 the president of the Canadian Life and Health Insurance Association (CLHIA), Alastair Fernie, warned that governments must perform radical surgery on health care to help solve Canada's debt crisis. Insurers, he said, could do their part by assisting governments to find services that "can and should" be covered by the private sector, including workers' compensation. "I believe that Canadians are still not getting the message that sacrifices will have to be made [to solve the debt crisis]," Fernie said, pointing in particular to "the younger generations" that had grown used to "getting things free."[7]

If "getting things free," including health care, was responsible for a litany of ills ranging from deficits to wait lists, paying for health-care services on the open market was seen as the cure. Insurers were not merely passive observers of federal and provincial initiatives, but were also actively involved in the development of domestic policies that would benefit their industry and support a thriving market for privately insured health services. Delisting medically unnecessary services from public health plans was one such policy that assisted the efforts of the private sector to convince Canadians that they must have those very same unnecessary services.

While many Canadians viewed delisting as a threat to universality, the private insurance industry described it as a "boon," predicting "the potential for millions of dollars of new business." In 1994, the CLHIA, which inherited the mantle of the CHIA, observed that five years earlier it had typically notified members that provincial governments had "added this or that benefit, so you're no longer needed to provide coverage." But a "totally different economic environment" in the mid-1990s meant the CLHIA could send out more cheerful notices advising members of recently delisted benefits they could now offer customers.[8]

Since the mid-1970s, Canadian insurers have aggressively pursued customers beyond their home borders, especially in the United States and, more recently, Asia, in order to increase premium income. Between 1975 and 1992, domestic premium revenues paid to Canadian life and health insurers increased by 470 percent, but revenues earned outside Canada increased by 1200 percent. By the mid-1990s, over 43 percent of premium income earned by Canadian life insurers originated outside the country, with several of the largest companies collecting between 50 and 80 percent of their total premium income from the United States alone. This compares to only 5 percent earned by U.S.-based corporations from extraterritorial premiums, and 10 percent earned by Australian companies.

Publicly insured health care was only one reason for seeking opportunities abroad, and it was not the primary one. The Canadian market was saturated with insurance products of every description by the late 1980s, and the country was second only to Japan in the number of people covered by life and health policies. Saturated markets precluded further growth in their home market, and with a growing percentage of premium income earned beyond their own borders, Canadian insurers identified expansion into the markets of other countries as a primary goal. Consequently, the Canadian health insurance industry was an early and enthusiastic proponent of free trade around the globe, and in this endeavour it had the unfailing support of federal Conservative and Liberal governments.

Canadian insurers identified strongly with the goals of free trade, especially the 1991 North American Free Trade Agreement, in part because these deals promised to open up the Mexican and U.S. markets. "Trade policy developments, such as NAFTA," said the CLHIA, "are custom made to fit the Canadian industry's outward thrust." But NAFTA also promised to bring increased pressure on Canada to emulate the deregulated insurance market of its southern neighbour and open up the domestic market to new investment opportunities for U.S. insurers.

Liberty Mutual and Ontario Blue Cross

Boston-based Liberty Mutual is one of many examples of this cross-border harmonization – or integration – of North America's insurance industry. U.S. insurers such as Aetna, Prudential Insurance, and Mutual of Omaha – all of whom spent a good part of the last two decades on the acquisition trail in the U.S. – have expanded their markets or acquired companies, in whole or in part, north of the forty-ninth parallel. All are positioning themselves to play a major role in the growing Canadian health industry.[9]

The purchase of Ontario Blue Cross (OBC) by Liberty International, a subsidiary of giant U.S. insurer Liberty Mutual, is probably the most prominent example of cross-border integration in the insurance industry to date. Founded in 1912 in Massachusetts, Liberty Mutual is one of the world's largest insurers, with 450 offices worldwide and more than 22,000 employees. Its net premium income in 1995 was almost $6 billion, and its assets – at more than $73 billion – are worth more than those of all Canadian health insurance companies combined. Its main line of business is workers' compensation and automobile insurance, but in recent years the company has expanded into the U.S. rehabilitation market, providing occupational health and safety programs to employers. The company's Canadian subsidiaries are run through Liberty International Canada, based in Toronto.

In August 1994 OBC announced it was looking for a partner "to fully realize its potential" to become Canada's largest health-benefits insurer. Any well-financed partner would do, said OBC officials, either domestic or foreign, and it was open to interested parties ranging from insurance to drug companies that could buy either some or all of the nonprofit health-benefits provider.

With over 2 million clients, and another 1.5 million Ontario residents not covered by benefits plans, OBC officials pointed to a growing and lucrative market for private insurers. And the speculation that annual private spending on health care in Ontario was set to rise from $3.6 billion in 1993 to between $5 billion and $8 billion by 1997 made the opportunity even more alluring. Liberty was definitely interested.[10]

OBC was wholly owned by Ontario's 220 publicly funded hospitals and managed by the Ontario Hospital Association. The OHA's former president, Dennis Timbrell, was well known to Liberty International. The decision to sell the nonprofit insurer was made in December 1993, according to Timbrell, who was appointed to Liberty's board of directors the following March. A month later he became chair of the board of directors of International Managed Health Care (IMHC), a rehabilitation company, rubbing elbows with Brian Johnston, Liberty Canada's president who also was on IMHC's board.

Shortly before Timbrell was appointed to Liberty's board, the OHA engaged investment bank ScotiaMcLeod to help find a buyer for OBC. The OHA advised Ontario's NDP government and the two Opposition parties of its intentions, but otherwise kept the pending sale out of the public spotlight. Timbrell, speaking on the record in early 1995, said the OHA had decided to sell its insurance arm so it could focus on "advocacy." In addition, the board of directors wanted OBC to become a managed care company, a proposition that required expensive new information systems and large amounts of investment capital unavailable to the nonprofit insurer.[11]

Liberty Canada CEO John McGlynn claimed his company first learned that OBC was for sale through a newspaper article in August 1994, but many observers voiced concern about Timbrell's relationship with the U.S. multinational and about what role he may have played in the negotiations between the two insurers. In mid-September, less than a month after reading about the sale, Liberty made a formal expression of interest. By December the two insurers announced they were entering into a "strategic alliance," an odd description for the outright takeover of OBC by the U.S. company. The acquisition opened up challenging new terrain for Liberty, which planned to use Canada "as a base for exporting managed care services world-wide." But for the people of Ontario it constituted the loss of a nonprofit alternative to the competitive, for-profit insurance industry, as well as the loss of a company in which the public had invested indirectly through Ontario's hospitals.[12]

Liberty's acquisition cost the company between $80 million and $100 million, plus another $888,000 in payouts to Timbrell and two other senior executives of the OHA. Johnston described OBC as a "natural fit" in the company's growing injury prevention, rehabilitation management, and occupational disability risk business. In addition, Liberty's global strategy of developing "exportable products," including its new kidnap and ransom insurance coverage, would be assisted by this acquisition. "We see the potential of providing OBC products, along with our technical capabilities, to international operators [in] emerging nations in Latin America and Asia," Johnston said. The only setback, said Liberty, was the decision by the Canadian Association of Blue Cross Plans to deny the new company the use of the prestigious Blue Cross trademark, which was bestowed only on nonprofit organizations. Thus, Liberty Health of Canada was born.[13]

Although the new owner had reassured the 650 employees of OBC that all of them "would retain their employment with OBC" and that they would "continue to receive staff benefits at current levels," in April 1996, 103 of them, layoff notices in hand, departed from the scene. "Our competitive position is jeopardized by staffing levels and work assignments no longer appropriate to the way we do business," explained Bill Wilkerson of Liberty Health. Management, he said, had planned all along to implement a major layoff. But employees could be forgiven if they had failed to understand that "retain ... employment" actually meant "major layoff" when the sale was finalized.[14]

Public protest throughout Ontario in response to the sale failed to convince the provincial government that the transfer of nonprofit OBC to a multinational corporate insurer should be blocked. In December 1994, Judy Darcy, president of the Canadian Union of Public Employees, demanded that the federal government halt the sale until a full public inquiry had been conducted to ascertain the consequences to the people of Ontario and of Canada. In a letter to Diane Marleau, then minister of health, Darcy expressed concern that "there may have been some profits going from the sale to the Ontario Hospital Association. We have grave concerns ... about how profits accumulated in the first place, and if so, who they belong to."

The Ontario Federation of Labour (OFL) also questioned Timbrell's role in the sale. Pointing to his position as both the president of OHA, which owned the insurer, and a member of Liberty International's board of directors, unions demanded an investigation of "the extent to which [Timbrell] will personally benefit from this sale." Julie Davis, secretary-treasurer of the OFL, urged the provincial government "to do everything in your power to see that the sale is halted pending a public enquiry." The OFL argued that OBC was funded from the $8 billion a year the provincial government allocated to the hospital sector and thus the sale, for all intents and purposes, was a major privatization of a public asset. "If the sale of Blue Cross to an American for-profit corporation proceeds, Canada takes another step towards privatization of its health care system," Davis wrote.[15]

Citizens' groups and several newspapers in Ontario backed the labour movement's demands for a public enquiry. The Canadian Health Coalition and the Council of Canadians both urged federal intervention in the sale, charging that failure to do so would "open the door to intrusion of for-profit companies in a big way." The Ottawa *Citizen* called for a "second opinion" on the takeover of OBC "by a U.S. company now also eyeing workers' compensation." Thomas Walkom, a columnist for the Toronto *Star*, kept up a steady barrage of criticism, asserting that Ontario's NDP government could block the sale "if it wanted." But what the provincial government wanted was not at all clear. Dismissing public concerns, which Finance Minister Floyd Laughren called "one of those strange tabloid crusades," the government said there was nothing it could do. "There appears to be nothing in existing laws that would allow us to stop [the sale], even if we wanted to," Laughren said. Nor did the government appear to have any appetite to introduce legislation that would give them the means to do so.[16]

The decision of the Ontario government to sit on its hands was perhaps no surprise. In 1990, when the NDP was elected with a broad mandate to introduce public auto insurance, the newly installed government had beat a quick retreat in the face of mounting pressure from the Canadian industry. The U.S. government, publicly urged on by American insurers, had added its weight to the question, threatening to challenge any such attempt under the Canada-U.S. Free Trade Agreement. When Liberty privately informed both the provincial and federal governments of its plans to acquire OBC in late 1993 (on the eve of yet another free trade deal) the provincial New Democrats appeared reluctant to take on such a large and powerful company.

The government's claim that it lacked the power to intervene roused little sympathy, especially among the province's hospital workers and patients. While the government said it could do nothing to protect Ontario's largest nonprofit insurer from a foreign takeover, it was able and willing to implement cuts in hospital funding and in the scope of benefits on the public health plan. It was able to reduce out-of-country medical coverage by $20 million, saying the savings were needed to help pay down the provincial deficit. These actions, coupled with a refusal to insure new medical procedures or provide coverage to foreign students, had helped increase the customer base of OBC, making the nonprofit insurer a more attractive investment for its new owner. If the provincial government could save money by cutting health care, many wondered, why couldn't they make sure that the $100 million netted by the OHA from the sale of OBC went into the provincial treasury?[17]

The role of NAFTA

The sale of OBC was made possible by the Canada-U.S. Free Trade Agreement and by NAFTA. These trade deals had removed a law imposing a 25 percent ceiling on foreign ownership in the insurance industry, a rule that ensured Canadians controlled the companies in the sector and that governments were able to regulate the industry. Canadian insurers did not view Liberty's acquisition as detrimental, since NAFTA was a two-way street: they were as busy in the U.S. market as U.S. insurers were in Canada's.

NAFTA's removal of restrictions on foreign ownership in the North American insurance market sparked an integration of the industries in the three countries covered by the agreement. What once were three nationally based industries in Canada, the U.S., and Mexico were merging into a single North American insurance industry that was carving up the continental market. The role of governments was being reduced to that of scout, keeping a close eye on the state of affairs in the insurance market in all three countries so that opportunities could be pointed out and then exploited on a "first come, first served" basis.

In 1991, for example, the U.S. consulate in Toronto observed steep increases in premiums charged by insurers selling supplementary health benefits to Canadian "snowbirds" who spent the winter in the more hospitable climes of Florida or Arizona. The information was duly noted and reported to U.S. insurance companies. "Many elderly

Canadians ... are reluctant to vacation in the U.S. because of the limits on their provincial insurance coverage" when they cross the border, said consular officer D. A. Wilson. Supplementary coverage, he added, had increased from $758 the previous year to $1400 for six months' worth of coverage. Opportunities for "additional U.S. health insurance companies in the Ontario market, and perhaps in other Canadian provincial markets as well" were abundant and "might also have the corollary effect of boosting U.S. winter tourism revenues."[18]

A few short years after NAFTA came into effect, the international boundaries that once governed the insurance industry were barely visible. In 1996 Aetna, a global health insurance company, declared it would "redefine the way health care is provided" in the United States, but its plan would be suitable for Canada, as well. In the same year, the company formed Aetna Health Management Canada Inc. and made its first acquisition in the Canadian health-care market with the purchase of Associative Rehabilitation Inc. (ARI) of London, Ontario. "Growing government cutbacks in health care, such as hospital closures," said Canadian CEO Ed Robinson, "have created business opportunities" for corporations in the health sector. Although Robinson said ARI was Aetna's first deal in Canada, it clearly would not be its last. "We intend to set the standard by which all Canadian health care companies will be measured," he said. The day after it announced the purchase of ARI, Aetna Canada director Ruth Grant was appointed to the board of trustees at Toronto's Hospital for Sick Children, giving the corporation a vantage point from which to closely monitor developments in the sector.[19]

Great West Life Assurance, owned by financial services and media giant Power Financial Corporation, was a Canadian player active in the U.S. insurance industry. Total premium income for the company was $8.5 billion for the first nine months of 1997, and its total assets were worth $44.8 billion. Most of Great West's premium income was earned in the U.S. market, where the company jumped wholeheartedly into the managed care revolution. In 1996, Great West formed One Health Plan in the United States, with the aim of developing a chain across the country. By the end of 1997 One Health Plan was well on its way, having established itself in eight states and become one of the largest "one-stop shopping" health centres in Colorado.[20]

Free trade was also expanding the variety of insurance products flooding into Canada. In 1995, North American Viatical Investments opened for business in Toronto with a U.S. partner, Mutual Benefits Corporation (MBC) of Fort Lauderdale, Florida. The two companies were marketing death benefits – the money paid out by a life insurance policy when the policy holder dies. In most cases this money goes to a spouse or children. Viatical investors buy rights to the death benefits of a policy held by an AIDS or cancer patient. The patient lists the investor as a beneficiary of his or her policy and in return the patient gets cash to purchase drugs and medical care. When the patient dies, the viatical investor will get back the original investment plus a premium of up to 42 percent. Said the *Financial Post*, "It's a US$400-million growth industry in the U.S., where late-stage AIDS and cancer victims need money to pay for medical care." AIDS patients were a better investment because their life expectancy was usually shorter than that of cancer patients and therefore the payout was quicker.

Viatical Investments' activities, described as "an adventure in the nature of trade" by a Revenue Canada official, are illegal in most Canadian provinces. Viatical's Canadian vice president, Bob Heward, said the company was selling its policies through 150 financial advisers across the country, giving Canadian investors access to the U.S. death benefits market. But Canada promised to be a tough market: there was less need for these types of investments, according to a representative of CLHIA, because of Canada's universal, publicly funded health-care system. Put more bluntly, Canadians did not have much incentive to invest in such ghoulish behaviour, nor did they have to, because lack of money was not a barrier to hospital and physician services under medicare.[21]

Integration in the North American insurance industry may provide economic benefits to Canadian companies, but it carries a high price tag for the country, including a substantial erosion of governments' legal rights to exercise regulatory and legislative control on behalf of citizens. According to Mickey Kantor, one of the chief U.S. negotiators at the NAFTA table and a close confidant of President Bill Clinton, free trade is not just about buying and selling goods and services, but about the export of "American values," as well, turning that country's passion for free enterprise and deregulation into a tool of U.S. foreign policy. "This is what we've meant … when we've declared that trade and economics are no longer a separate sphere from the rest of American foreign policy," said Kantor. "Anyone who doesn't see that these are inextricably connected hasn't stopped to look at what's happening."[22]

The interweaving of Canada's health-care system with that of the United States is not being done to bring a higher degree of equity and accessibility to the American people. Rather, the opposite is true: the imposition of a grossly inefficient and unjust system of market medicine prevalent in the U.S. is as much a part of NAFTA as the free flow of health-care goods and services back and forth across the border.

The Canadian health and insurance industries have undergone radical changes since medicare was introduced in the late 1960s. The alliance between the insurance industry and the medical profession provided both groups with a powerful voice during the early medicare debates and substantial influence over the kind of health-care system that developed during the decades that followed. The insurance industry's relationship with the medical profession during the years preceding medicare often was tense, with what were called "philosophical differences" between the two groups erupting from time to time. These differences revolved around the question of how – and whether – profits could justifiably be extracted from people who needed health care. Today these differences have all but disappeared. While physicians have long abandoned the health-insurance field, they have asserted their interests as entrepreneurs with businesses to run. The relationship between insurers and physicians now is based as much on a common political agenda as on developing their common business interests. Doctors see privately insured patients who bring in higher physician fees than public medicare, while insurers view doctors as custodians who determine how much, or how little, and what kind of medical care patients receive.

In the main, however, the insurance industry spends less time developing its relationships with doctors than it does securing more business-friendly national policies. These efforts were focussed on free trade and deregulation in the 1980s and on the so-called "managed care revolution" of the 1990s, which promised a significantly increased role for private insurers in how health care would be – or would not be – delivered. These efforts required alliances of a different kind. The emerging corporate health sector was a more powerful ally than physicians, and one that, like the insurance industry, was going global.

SIX

Health-Care Services: The Politics of Privatization

Privatization is occurring across the country, and throughout the health-care system, in both visible and invisible ways. On the surface, privatization appears to be the result of other priorities, such as government decisions to fight the deficit by cutting back what is spent on social programs. But while corporate and political leaders may not state the obvious, for many privatization is a political objective in and of itself.

Privatization, efficiency, and globalization

Privatization as a goal is linked to the federal and many provincial governments' desire to create an export-oriented economy and to attract foreign investment. Foreign investors (in particular those based in the United States) have expressed a strong interest in Canada's health-care sector – or health industry, as it is described in the marketplace – for many years. As U.S. health investors have increased their presence in the domestic market, Canada's health industry has become increasingly integrated with that of the rest of North America.

North America's health-service, medical devices, supplies, and distribution markets are larger than the automobile, steel, and transportation sectors combined. But health is an industry dominated by corporations based in the United States, which has the most extensive private health industry in the world, one that leads the globe both in terms of size and scope. In 1996, for example, the annual revenues of Columbia/HCA, the world's largest hospital corporation, exceeded the annual income of every provincial government in Canada except Québec and Ontario.

About 750,000 people work in Canada's health sector. Between 70 and 75 percent of health care is delivered in nonprofit clinics and institutions, most of which are hospitals. More than 25 percent of health services are delivered in the for-profit sector by 2500 firms – a figure that doesn't include doctors, 64 percent of whom are private, fee-for-service entrepreneurs. Ninety percent of these firms are small or medium-sized, employing more than 150,000 people nationwide and commanding revenues of between $3 and $3.5 billion a year. Another 800 companies in Canada, with 20,000 employees, produce and supply support services for health-care appliances and devices, part of a world market worth $93 billion annually, $2.5 billion of which is spent by Canadian consumers.[1]

There are about 250 large corporations, most of them U.S.-based, involved in Canada's health-care sector. These provide a range of goods and services from insurance, information technology, and food to drugs, advice, and home care. Governments used to regulate the investments of corporations across the economy, especially in areas like health care, to ensure that such investments demonstrated a public good. Now, however, the objectives of government and the corporate sector are indistinguishable. These include consolidation in the health industry, reductions in the size and scope of the public sector (including reductions in public health-care expenditures), privatization, and a strengthened role for Canadian companies in the global economy.

To achieve these domestic goals and penetrate international markets, many large corporations have concluded that Canada's health industry must achieve greater consolidation to eliminate the waste and duplication (and even "triplication") that characterize the country's current fragmented market. The federal government fully concurs with this perspective and has made it a priority to assist the industry in attracting both domestic and foreign investment to finance the growth and concentration of Canadian health companies. "Promoting Canadian companies as global health-keepers," said Industry Canada in 1997, "is the main objective driving the strategies and plans" of the government for the medical devices, pharmaceutical, and health-services sectors. "Governments have an important role to play in setting the business climate at home."

These strategies are being developed jointly with Canada's health industries, business associations, and provincial governments. There are no trade unions or employee groups at the table, no organizations representing patients nor representatives of the many groups across the country working to protect and strengthen publicly funded health services.[2]

The federal government officially embraced foreign investment in Canada's health industry when it signed the Canada-U.S. Free Trade Agreement and, two years later, NAFTA. These and other "trade liberalization" deals have been designed to enable money to flow freely across international boundaries without restraint or the interference of national criteria. Rules requiring that investments provide a benefit to the people of Canada may be deemed a "barrier" to investment, and governments that impose such rules may be subject to stiff penalties. From Ottawa's perspective, foreign direct investment provides small and medium-sized Canadian companies with access to the capital only large global corporations can provide. This capital, according to the federal government, is sorely lacking in the domestic market. Foreign investment is also viewed as an integral plank in the government's privatization strategies.

In a paper published by the World Bank in 1996 and funded by the Canadian International Development Agency (CIDA), an arm of the Ministry of Foreign Affairs, the objectives of government and the role of foreign investment in privatization were clearly and frankly spelled out. Privatization, the paper stated, enables governments to "fund other expenditures, reduce taxation, reduce the public sector deficit or repay domestic and foreign public debt," all goals set by the Canadian government during the past decade. Sectors dominated by public enterprises are isolated from international competition and, at the same time, suffer from a "scarcity of domestic entrepreneurs and investors" who can assist in efforts to privatize. For these reasons, foreign investors are vital partners in Canada's privatization initiatives, and their exclusion will doom such initiatives to failure, and inhibit the development of a thriving private sector.[3]

Foreign investment also brings other benefits, according to the paper, including reductions in the size and scope of the public sector and in the influence of "pressure groups" such as trade unions and opposition political parties. Foreign investments also minimize "the possibility for a successor government to reverse the privatization process," since investors can enlist the aid of their own governments in bringing pressure on the host country. But because "privatization is politically dangerous," governments must ensure that "various interest groups" are excluded from the process. "Of particular importance is the exclusion of any party" that wants to protect the public's investment, "especially the workforce, the management and [relevant government] ministries." It is hardly surprising, therefore, that the Canadian people have not been present during Ottawa's consultations with global companies regarding future directions for health care.[4]

Federal policymakers, led by those in Industry Canada and External Affairs, believe that by linking Canadian health companies to foreign multinationals they are paving the way to global markets where "very substantial amounts of money are being spent on health care." But Canadian companies face a number of obstacles when they try to export health services and products: the nation's health industry is fragmented; it is small in size, with limited resources to fund expansion and acquisitions; it lacks export experience. Multinationals, on the other hand, offer global experience and competitive advantages that provide their Canadian partners with "the potential for growth and the opportunity to become less dependent upon the domestic market." And since few firms in the domestic health sector have "the critical mass and financial resources to continually market their services abroad," a growing chorus in Industry Canada says, there must be "increased cooperation and collaboration between the private sector and public sector, including its publicly funded health care institutions," such as hospitals. Such collaboration provides a funnel through which public funds can be channelled to under-resourced private companies.[5]

Canada's export focus for the health industry has necessarily influenced domestic policies for the sector. "While notable exceptions exist, in most cases domestic success precedes success abroad," the Ontario government's Health Industries Committee concluded in 1994. The group's views dovetailed neatly with those of Industry Canada. "To have the effective launching pad it needs," the committee said, the "health industries sector must expand its share of its own home market. Steps must be taken to ensure that, as in other countries, the domestic market supports the development of globally competitive companies."[6]

Federal and provincial policies leading to decreased hospital services or outright hospital closures, therefore, complement goals and strategies designed to strengthen public-private partnerships in the domestic health market. The closure of hospitals and hospital outpatient departments is creating a vacuum increasingly filled, not by locally based, nonprofit providers, but by subsidiaries of global, U.S.-based corporations.

The Columbia Health Care story

Columbia Health Care Inc. (not to be confused with U.S.-based Columbia/HCA), for example, is considered a stellar success story by many corporate and government leaders who support privatization. Founded in 1978 in Kelowna, B.C., by psychiatrist Dr. Charles Gregory, Columbia provided rehab services for patients in the region suffering from chronic back pain. Many of the small company's referrals came from the Insurance Corporation of B.C. (ICBC), the provincial auto insurer, and from the Workers' Compensation Board (WCB).

In 1987, at the invitation of the Ontario WCB, Gregory opened a second clinic in Toronto, where opportunities were opening up in the workers' compensation rehabilitation area. But Gregory appears not to have been interested in building a corporate empire. In 1990, when he sold Columbia for $1 million to William Brown, a drugstore and phar-maceutical executive, there were only twenty-five employees working in the two clinics established by the founder.[7]

Brown, however, was an empire builder. Prior to his takeover of Columbia, he had served a three-year stint as president and CEO of Medis Health & Pharmaceutical Services, a health-services and drug distributor with 1300 employees and annual revenues of over $1 bil-lion. Immediately after acquiring Columbia, Brown began combing Bay Street for investors willing to inject the cash he would need to expand Canada-wide. He raised $10 million in venture capital funding from Canada's largest health corporation, MDS Inc., and Manulife Financial, the Prudential Insurance Corporation of America, and the Ontario Hydro pension fund.

The introduction of no-fault auto insurance in Ontario in 1991 allowed private insurers to offer auto accident victims suffering severe head injuries up to $1 million for treatment. The private rehab market took off, and Columbia's fortunes improved considerably. Within three years, Columbia was operating eighteen clinics with 180 employees and annual revenues of $11 million – and was casting an eager eye in the direction of the disability and workers' comp rehabilitation business.

Rehab services are a vital step in the health-care chain, assisting injured patients in recovery and teaching them how to avoid further injury. By the mid-1990s, rehab services had been identified as a "mar-ket niche" by many companies anxious to cash in on privatization as cutbacks rippled through the sector.[8]

Funding for rehabilitation services comes from a variety of sources in Canada: public and private health plans, public and private auto insurers, workers' compensation boards, and direct patient user fees. Rehab services delivered on an outpatient basis by a hospital are included in the hospital's global budget allocation, and user fees are prohibited, but many provinces have establish a fee structure to pay for services provided by private rehabilitation therapists. These thera-pists are able to charge the patient or the patient's supplementary insurer, an additional, fixed user fee.

Brown boasted that "none of [Columbia's] revenues come from medicare or the government; we're strictly in the private sector." This fact would have made the company almost completely unique in Canada ... if it had been true. In British Columbia, unions representing hospital-based physio and occupational therapists and rehab aides had lobbied the provincial government to establish guidelines ensuring both the Crown corporation ICBC and the Workers' Compensation Board referred patients to publicly funded hospitals instead of private companies such as Columbia. But the closure of hospital outpatient services and the growth of private rehab companies to replace, or in some cases displace, hospital clinics across the country were making such government directives – where they existed – potentially harmful to the public. Patients covered by public insurance plans often had no choice but use Columbia's facilities, and Columbia did not refuse to accept the public payment that came with them.[9]

Brown was anxious to acquire a larger share of the workers' comp pie, and in his pitch to employers he asserted that businesses could save money by referring workers injured on the job to Columbia. Funded by private-sector money, Columbia offered services ranging from vocational coaching and community reintegration to speech and therapy programs designed to restore mobility and function to disabled workers. In addition to referrals from employers, physicians, and quasi-public or public institutions, Columbia targeted two "market segments" it had identified as growth areas: injured workers and auto accident victims (and their lawyers). The opening of a neuro-rehabilitation centre in Toronto early in 1994, coupled with Columbia's rapid growth-by-acquisition and its partnerships with larger corporations, helped establish the company as one of Canada's largest rehabilitation service providers. With the private – and privately insured – home, rehab, and long-term care markets opening up, Columbia was well-positioned to meet its corporate goals.[10]

The capital infusion Columbia received in 1990 had not come without the requisite trail of strings, one of which gave MDS 42 percent of shares in, and effective control of, the company, while another 10 percent of shares went to Manulife. In addition, two MDS executives sat as directors on Columbia's board, while the two companies shared a 50-50 partnership in the Ottawa-based Canadian Injury Recovery Clinic. In 1995, Columbia's Board of Directors, headed by Richard

Lockie of MDS, approved the sale of the rehab company to New Mexico-based Sun Healthcare Group, Inc. for $8.7 million. Columbia was now part of somebody else's corporate empire.[11]

Sun Healthcare and the Canadian market

Sun Healthcare was the creation of Andrew Turner, an outspoken opponent of public-sector involvement in the health industry. Dubbed "Andy the Dynamic" by the *New Mexico Business Journal*, Turner's legend included the requisite story about his humble beginnings in the health business, made possible when his church pastor asked Turner to take over management of the congregation's nursing home in 1974. Within ten years, Turner and two partners had founded the Hillhaven Corporation and, later, the Horizon Health Care Corporation, both of Tacoma, Washington. Horizon relocated to the more hospitable climes of New Mexico and went on to become the largest rehab services company in the U.S., merging with fellow rehab giant HealthSouth in 1997.

In 1989 Turner took seven unprofitable nursing homes, his share of the original company, and formed the Sun Healthcare Group, now one of the largest nursing home companies in the U.S., with long-term, rehabilitation and pharmacy services divisions in forty-eight states. When Sun acquired Columbia Health Care Inc. in 1995, it had 161 long-term and nursing home facilities, nearly 17,000 beds, 28,000 employees, revenues of US$1.3 billion – and an appetite for going abroad.[12]

Sun's entry into Canada reflected the company's tentative expansion into the outpatient rehab business. In the United States, not-for-profit rehabilitation providers were struggling to keep their heads above water in a pool increasingly dominated by large companies able to offer an array of physio, occupational and speech therapy, respiratory, and psychological counselling services on a contract basis to nonacute-care providers. Services provided outside of the acute-care hospital sector in the U.S. were in chaos and in need of some kind of rationalization. Both public and private payers were demanding lower costs, and hospitals responded with the introduction of tightened admissions criteria and decreased inpatient stays. As a consequence, other levels of care were emerging or growing outside the hospitals. In the rehab sector alone there were 204 inpatient hospitals operating at the end of 1996, 130 of which were under one corporate roof after the Horizon-HealthSouth merger. Most of the remainder were nonprofit, stand-alone hospitals scattered coast to coast. There were also 3200 private physiotherapy practices, 1122 outpatient rehab centres, 1498 diagnostic imaging centres, 1651 outpatient surgery centres, and 135 occupational health clinics – none of which were under the control of the major chains. It was a fragmented, $16 billion industry, and a prime candidate for consolidation.[13]

Nursing home chains, caught up in the shifting terrain of the U.S. health-care sector, were becoming more concentrated in fewer hands. Many were integrating their rehab services with new levels of service called assisted living or sub-acute care, a level that catered to those too sick to go home but not sick enough to stay in hospital. Sun's rapid acquisition of nursing homes and outpatient rehab clinics helped establish the company as one of the largest nursing home chains in the nation, with a complementary network of support services for its facilities. "The timing [of acquisitions] has to do with Wall Street's enthusiasm for nursing-home stocks," said Turner, an explanation that would dispel notions that the company was intent on filling a need for health-care service. And timing was everything: while the stock market smiled on nursing home companies in 1994, eighteen months later uncertainty about Washington's plans for Medicare funding caused trading levels to fall by 40 percent.[14]

Sun's rapid expansion across the United States also was fuelled by an equally rapid growth in revenues, a generous portion of which came from the public purse – in fact, only 25 percent of its net revenues came from private payers in 1995. The rest of Sun's U.S. profits could be traced to Medicaid, a public insurance program for poor people, and Medicare, a federal program for the elderly and disabled. With the establishment of several new divisions, designed to serve both its own subsidiaries as well as nonaffiliated nursing homes and long-term care facilities, Sun's growth strategy became more focussed and disciplined. Increasingly, its acquisitions were strategically designed to support Sun as a multinational long-term care provider with a diverse portfolio of complementary services, including medical and equipment supplies, drugs, and therapy services, the latter composed of contract, outpatient, and temporary staffing subsidiaries. As the company's position in the U.S. health industry attained a degree of stability, it set its sights on countries undergoing privatization in their health-care sectors, namely Britain, Australia, and Canada.[15]

By the end of 1996, after a series of buy-outs in England, Sun was the second largest operator of nursing and residential support facilities in the United Kingdom. A pharmaceutical subsidiary Suncript was set up to serve the growing number of Sun nursing homes in England, a project that necessitated a parallel buying spree of pharmacies throughout the country. An investment six months later in Alpha Healthcare Ltd., the second largest private hospital operator in New South Wales, Australia, gave Sun "an opportunity … to leverage its clinical expertise in an emerging healthcare marketplace," according to Turner, meaning that profits could be pried out of the publicly subsidized Australian health system. "This investment will enable us to learn more about the Australian marketplace," he said, which in turn would give Sun experience in how to operate in the international health-care arena.[16]

Sun hoped that its November 1995 acquisition of Columbia Health Care and its nineteen rehab clinics in Ontario, Alberta, and British Columbia would provide the company with a foothold in the Canadian market, particularly as governments moved health services into the for-profit sector. The buy-out, said Turner, "builds on the international growth strategy we began earlier this year in the United Kingdom." He added that with the "reliable revenue stream from our UK operation, we believe the timing is appropriate for us to take the next step in developing our international goals." Sun's U.K. revenue stream undoubtedly improved its standing, but its acquisitions in Canada were financed largely by a revolving line of credit at a bank in Texas. Although Turner promised to bring the expertise Sun had gained in the U.S. to "new markets abroad," the company chose not to apply its acquired skills in Canada's long-term care sector, an area in which it would confront some formidable domestic contenders, including giant Ontario-based Extendicare. The fact that Canadians historically were highly proficient at not only designing rehab services, but in making them accessible as well, may have been a consideration in Sun's boardroom. But it was the potential for profits in a market undergoing rapid privatization, as well as the country's abundance of skill and experience, that made Columbia a ripe target for acquisition.[17]

Less than a year after the purchase, Columbia could attest to the advantages it had gained from Sun's expertise. Columbia's strength, Brown had said in 1994, was its ability to "move people from the liability side of the human balance sheet over to the asset side," a task that was made easier with Sun's financial backing. Sun made good on its promise to provide up to $12 million a year to fund Columbia's acquisitions. In 1996, seven new clinics were added to the fold, including "3270262 Canada, Inc.," an outpatient physiotherapy and occupational services company, and Aqua Rehabilitation, Inc., for $4 million. The $4.1 million purchase of International Managed Health Care, the troubled Liberty International subsidiary with nine clinics, in August 1996 signalled Columbia's – and Sun's – commitment to "move swiftly to seize opportunities in the burgeoning private health industry" in Canada. Sun Healthcare, said Warren McInteer, in charge of the company's mergers and acquisitions strategy, was "interested in the transition in the Canadian marketplace from the public sector to the private sector." No doubt it was also interested in Columbia's 1995/96 revenues, which Brown said exceeded $35 million.[18]

Despite his enthusiasm for American dollars, Brown, now Sun's lead hand at Columbia, was touchy about suggestions he might be selling out to a U.S. investor. "I have no wish to draw focus to it [Sun's ownership]," Brown told a reporter. "I don't want people to think this is an American company." But if Columbia was "very much the same company" it was before Sun's acquisition, it was now "being fuelled using U.S. currency," Brown said, and this money would enable him to aggressively "grow" his enterprise "at approximately 50 per cent per annum." By the end of 1996 Columbia's strategy seemed to be working: there were now more than thirty outpatient rehab clinics in its lineup, and with privatization escalating as federal and provincial cuts to health care continued, the future definitely looked promising.[19]

Certainly Andrew Turner should have been pleased by the accelerated pace of privatization in his new field of operation. In an interview in April 1996 he was asked what he saw as the proper role of government in the health-care system. "The government should butt out," Turner responded. "If that happened, market forces would quickly resolve the problems of the industry." If this sounded odd coming from a company that derived 75 percent of its revenues from the public purse, it wasn't. "We have an obligation to provide health care for poor people," Turner explained, "but it should be managed health care under rules provided by the private sector." If the government left things to the private sector, quality would improve, Turner said, because the "marketplace would close poor operators ... people would shop," and providers who didn't offer the best care "would be out of business."[20]

In late 1997 Sun reorganized its Canadian holdings, consolidating and relocating the headquarters of Columbia's western operations to Calgary and appointing Tom Saunders as president. Saunders had a history in Alberta's for-profit rehab market as the head of Western Occupational Rehabilitation Centre in Calgary, a company he sold to Columbia. The same year, Saunders became a director of the controversial Calgary-based Health Resources Group (HRG), Canada's first for-profit hospital. Worried Albertans and Opposition critics in the legislature said Saunders' involvement with an American company could lead to Sun's takeover of HRG. William Brown, meanwhile, departed the Sun empire, reappearing as an executive of Aetna Canada, another U.S. company that was expanding its Canadian rehab business. Sun claimed its reorganization of Columbia Health Care was undertaken "in response to increasing pressures across Canada, by both private and government payers, to lower costs and improve operating efficiencies in the delivery of healthcare services." The company said it expected to continue to play an active role in the Canadian health industry.[21]

Legislating the second tier

The takeover of much of Canada's rehabilitative services by a multinational, U.S.-based corporation – and one that is vocally hostile to government involvement in the provision of health services – is considered a "success story" by many public policymakers across the country. It is the story of a small B.C. company that grew through acquisitions and mergers and that consequently was integrated into the North American operations of an experienced global corporation. But for the Canadian people, such integration is not a good-news story. On the contrary, it underscores the threat to universal access posed by Ottawa's privatization and reduced funding strategies. And it points to the failure of the federal government's promotion of "Canadian companies as global health-keepers," a strategy that promises to undermine, not promote, Canadian ownership and control in a vital sector of the economy.

Although Ottawa has declared its commitment to medicare and the principles of the Canada Health Act, these pronouncements are contradicted by deep cuts in federal funding and the strengthening of policies specifically designed to assist corporations investing in the sector. Not only is Ottawa funding corporate health initiatives that often consume hundreds of millions of dollars, it is also fostering strategic cross-border alliances that result in private monopolies. These corporate monopolies – or "group synergies" – enable firms to "combat intense international competition resulting from the globalization of the world economy." And in case anyone thought that such relationships violated Canada's competition laws, "the government stance today is radically different: most business alliances are now seen as beneficial to the economy and are being promoted by various policy initiatives."[22]

Deficits and globalization are the main factors cited by governments in the "tough" decisions they make about decreasing overall public expenditures. Within this framework, health spending can be placed in opposition to other pressing and publicly funded needs from education and highway construction to child poverty and salaries for public employees. "You have to choose between health care and anti-poverty programs," governments seem to be saying, "but you can't have both."

Funding reductions for health are supported by the business sector because they skew the overall distribution of wealth in favour of those who already have wealth, and because such reductions ease pressure on governments to seek revenues in the form of corporate taxes. Between 1986 and 1997 spending reductions for health totalled approximately $37 billion, and were paralleled by huge decreases in the amount of tax revenue collected from corporations. Although the corporate sector is fond of decrying the amount of money it contributes to public coffers, corporate tax payments fell from 17 percent of total tax revenues in the mid-1980s to less than 9 percent today. (Compare this to the situation in the 1950s when corporate taxes made up approximately 52 percent of tax revenues.)[23]

Ironically, as corporations pay less in taxes for health care, government cutbacks have significantly expanded the role these corporations play in the major decisions affecting every aspect of health care and, therefore, of Canadians' health. Decreased public funding is increasing the control insurers and employers have over the behaviour of the workforce – they are now able to dictate what prescription drugs workers take, what services they receive and how doctors treat them when they're ill, the duration of sick time they are allowed, and how workers "manage" their chronic conditions. This is happening even as employers shift a greater portion of the cost of insurance premiums to individual workers.

The private sector has viewed government reductions in funding for health care as a mixed blessing. Both large and small businesses have criticized what they describe as a downloading of costs to employer-sponsored supplementary health plans that cover some 20 million Canadian workers and their dependants. Small and medium-sized companies in particular have felt the squeeze as their insurance premiums increased, necessitating elaborate strategies for further cost shifting to employees. But for large corporations, which were (and are) the chief proponents of funding cuts to health and social programs, the benefits have far outweighed the disadvantages. For big business, the shift in who controls the purse strings is, by and large, good news.

The Canadian Medical Association and its provincial divisions have warned Canadians about what they refer to as "passive privatization." This threatens to create a second tier of medicine for the wealthy, the CMA warns, who can afford the highest quality and most up-to-date medical treatment anywhere at any time. But the CMA – in keeping with its historical position – has not fought against "two-tiered medicine" in the era of medicare cutbacks. Rather, it has demanded that

Canadians face up to the limitations of public funding and force policymakers to allow "alternative sources of funding," a veiled reference to the private insurance industry. A second tier should be legislated and defined formally, the CMA asserts, and not created by stealth.

If funding cuts have shifted control over health care from the public to the private sector, mergers and foreign investment in the health and insurance industries are shifting control to the head offices of multinational corporations. As smaller Canadian-owned health companies, such as Columbia Health Care, merge with U.S.-based global corporations, they are able to tap into larger pools of capital and use a broader array of technical and other resources they need to survive. In exchange, the decisions that affect the private health industry in Canada increasingly are made in global headquarters south of the border, decreasing the ability of Canadian managers to implement "made in Canada" strategies. Of forty pharmaceutical companies surveyed by Industry Canada in 1996, for example, twenty were subsidiaries of multinational corporations. Of these twenty companies, fourteen felt that they had little if any autonomy in deciding which markets to target with which products. Increasingly, said the group of fourteen, such decisions were made "strictly" by their head offices.[24]

The priority for subsidiaries in the era of globalization is to "add value" to the parent corporation, rather than to address the needs of customers in the Canadian market. "Fundamentally," observed Julian Birkenshaw, an academic at the University of Western Ontario, "the multinational subsidiary has no rights to any business activities other than those that are focused on selling in the local market," and these activities are undertaken exclusively to enhance the profit margins of the parent company. Companies that fail to provide a return on investment are disciplined by the market, which cares very little about whether or not local community interests are being served.[25]

Federal and provincial governments have concluded that to successfully implement their export-focussed objectives and attract foreign direct investment in the health industry there must be changes in the domestic policies affecting the sector. When the Alberta government closed Calgary's two city hospitals, for example, the Health Resources Group stepped in to fill the vacuum, with $2 million in its pocket from the Canadian Medical Discovery Fund, an investment fund jointly run by MDS, the Medical Research Council of Canada, and other private health investors. Provincial funding cuts to hospitals also have sparked a search for alternative sources of revenue in for-profit enterprises shared 50-50 with large, global corporations. Such enterprises meet Ottawa's goal of "partnering" publicly funded institutions and private companies. Funding cuts have also led hospitals to seek "efficiencies" in outsourcing – despite warnings from numerous U.S. studies that show this may not be an avenue to saving money. It is, however, a way to channel public money to large corporations. Hospital cuts to outpatient services ranging from rehabilitation to diagnostic and X-ray services have supported, both directly and indirectly, the expansion of for-profit companies, many of which appear destined (if not anxious) to adapt their nationality to the demands of the global marketplace.

The privatization thrust of Canada's health policy is creating new types of consortiums funded with large doses of public money. The Canadian Institute for Health Information (CIHI), which bills itself as a private, not-for-profit organization, was formed to manage the country's health data bases and registries. These services used to be provided by Statistics Canada, Health Canada, and the Hospital Medical Records Institute and were available as public information.

CIHI is funded by large corporations such as IBM, Hewlett-Packard, SmartHealth (a subsidiary of the Royal Bank of Canada), SHL Systemhouse (a subsidiary of U.S.-based telecommunications giant, MCI), and several hospitals working in partnership with the corporate sector and other Canadian- and U.S.-based companies. The head of CIHI is Michael Decter, Canadian vice president of APM, Inc., a U.S.-based firm that offers advice to hospitals about how to partner with the corporate sector. The information CIHI collects – on health services and expenditures, and financial, statistical, and clinical data – is provided to anyone who can afford the hefty fees. For an annual membership fee of between $1000 and $5000, companies can "influence the establishment of national health informatics standards" and network with national and international experts in the health-care business. In this way, information that is vital to influencing the direction of Canada's health system has been removed from public sources and reorganized to benefit corporate investors.

However, information about those corporate investors – never easy to obtain from public sources in Canada – is more difficult to come by than it used to be. After the election of the federal Liberals in 1991, Canadian corporations doing business in the U.S. urged the new prime minister, Jean Chretien, to lobby Washington, D.C., for a change in the regulations that required the information they filed with the U.S. Securities and Exchange Commission (SEC) to be publicly available. Many Canadian researchers used the SEC to obtain information about, for example, salaries paid to corporate executives in Canada. Researchers turned to the SEC because this and other information about Canadian companies was unavailable from public Canadian sources. This was patently unfair, Canadian companies asserted, and Chretien agreed. And so, apparently, did the U.S. government, which amended the regulations so that Canadian-based companies would no longer be required to file information about their Canadian activities with the SEC.

Public money, private profits

Corporations and governments believe that "strategic partnering" between public and private sectors will offer new sources of funding for health-care institutions, at the same time providing health companies with access to pools of expertise and a highly trained workforce. Collaborations among health companies, governments, university- and hospital-based researchers, and hospitals would put some "synergetic" sparkle into the ailing health system. "The game is changing, and so is the playing field," David MacKinnon of the Ontario Hospital Association told a conference on public-private partnering in 1996. The private sector, he said, already is "guiding our hospital system," where "many members of hospital boards and a disproportionate number of Board chairs are business people." Such partnerships are "imperative," he added, and "the time for action has arrived."[26]

The growth of Canada's private health industry is framed by federal policies designed to exploit the opportunities of the global marketplace. Provincial governments are also working hard to attract "high tech" health and pharmaceutical investors, hoping to steer their economies away from a traditional resource or agricultural base by luring health, drug, and information technology companies with a variety of incentives. Like the companies they court, provinces have their eyes on the global marketplace, despairing of Canada's small population, which stubbornly insists on universal medicare. Health-care companies, for their part, are sizing up the provincial landscape, looking for "prime investment sites" in which to do business and avoid paying their fair share of taxes.

One province that has worked hard to develop a welcoming infrastructure in hopes of transforming its economic dependence on farm production to an economy based on high-tech health care is Manitoba. "It's taking plough shears and turning them into health products," said Nigel Lilley of Manitoba's Health Industry Development Initiative (HIDI) in 1996. Revenues in the province's health-industries sector had grown by nearly 1300 percent since 1984, when only four companies with combined earnings of $25 million were operating. A decade later, that number had grown to 103: 13 pharmaceutical companies with combined revenues of $188 million, and 90 medical device companies with revenues of $105 million. This growth, boasted Lilley, had created the third largest health industries sector in Canada, thanks to the generous financial and political support of the provincial Ministry of Industry, Trade and Tourism.[27]

Manitoba's arms and purse were open, and the government's efforts to establish the province as a leader in the health industry were assisted by the federal government's Western Economic Diversification (WED) program. Although Manitoba was tackling the deficit by reducing funding to the public health-care sector, its Industrial Opportunities Program was able to scrape together $2.67 million in November 1994 to help a new company, National Healthcare Manufacturing Corp. (NHMC), get off the ground. Ottawa topped up the province's financial assistance to NHMC with another $1.95 million.

In early 1997 the WED program joined with the Royal Bank in a joint $20 million investment loan program to "strengthen the growth and export potential of small health industry businesses in Western Canada." Dr. Jon Gerrard, secretary of state for WED and a Liberal MP from Manitoba, was enthusiastic about the growth potential of the private health-care industry despite the constant reassurances his government had given residents about its commitment to public health care. The global medical industry, Gerrard said, was worth hundreds of billions of dollars and "worldwide," he enthused, "it's probably going to double in the next five years." Canada needed to grab a greater share of the pie.

NHMC agreed, using government loans to develop "the world's first and only" advanced robotics production facility to assemble, package, and market medical and surgical products. "Nobody's done this in the world before," said Reg Ebbeling, chair and director of NHMC and former managing partner of HIDI. NHMC was developing an automated production line whose output hopefully was heading south into the estimated $2 billion U.S. market for medical/surgical kits and patient-care trays.

The company's growth was fuelled by "an aggressive sales, marketing and acquisitions strategy to capture a significant market share in the rapidly expanding multi-billion dollar medical device industry." But NHMC was not promising jobs to Manitobans. Far from it: the company was planning to become a leader "in displacing traditional hospital and distribution activities" – and in displacing well-paying, unionized jobs. NHMC's products, acquired from a number of manufacturers, were assembled on its robotic assembly line in Winnipeg and distributed to hospitals, outpatient surgery centres, dental and medical clinics, long-term care facilities, and home-care providers. The company's robotics technology, it repeatedly boasted, gave its packaging arm "the speed and accuracy necessary" to produce "at lower cost than the competition who manually assemble and package their kits and trays."

NHMC, structured as a "hub and spoke" operation with five divisions, pursued partnership arrangements with Manitoba hospitals that went "beyond the classic hospital and distributor relationship." For NHMC, the partnership with publicly funded providers – or rather with public funds – focussed "on how the partners can complement each other to manage the risks together throughout the health care system," in particular in the perilous waters of the private market. If the company failed in the competitive fast lane, it was comforting to know that the public would "share the risk." It was also a great comfort to know that the public, entirely unaware of its contribution, would not be clamouring for a share of the rewards.

The services offered to hospitals by NHMC included a computerized storage and retrieval system for medical records, X-rays, and files; a linen and laundry service; a copier centre; biohazardous waste pickup and disposal; and biomedical services. The company's structure, said NHMC, was designed for the integrated health-care system of the future and was the next step in the evolution of health-care distribution services. And it was all being done with fewer than twenty-five employees, something that might have been difficult for the Manitoba government to explain after so enthusiastically backing this golden opportunity to enhance job creation and the province's economy.

NHMC may not have been contributing a substantial boost to the provincial economy, but its own bottom line was very healthy. "Manitoba is less than half of one per cent of what we're going to do," said Bob Jackson, the company's vice president and CEO. In September 1996 the company reported it had netted $672,738 in sales during the previous three months, up almost 22 percent from the same period a year earlier. Its target for the upcoming year was between $10 million and $15 million, a goal it was confident it would reach.

But if any Manitobans had known enough about the company to ask how much of that money was being reinvested in their province, they would have learned it was very little. All of NHMC's strategies were designed to support acquisitions and alliances outside the province – or, as explained by the company, to facilitate "faster penetration into the United States market." The opening of a 72,000 square foot manufacturing facility in Winnipeg – "the geographic and time zone centre of North America" – in July 1995 was followed by several acquisitions that expanded NHMC's reach to Chicago, San Antonio, Toronto, Vancouver, and Sweden within two years. "The health care industry is currently undergoing significant transformation and reform," the company said in 1997, "driven, not by legislation, but by major purchasers of health care." Having received the support of both Manitoba and Ottawa for its ambitious undertakings, the National Healthcare Manufacturing Corporation was going global, and if it followed the plans laid out by the federal government, it would soon be merging with a larger, more experienced company. Manitobans would be lucky to see fifty jobs in return for their hospitality.[28]

SEVEN

The Market Gets Another Leg Up

Canadian governments and health corporations promoting the integration of North America's health industry are getting much of their leadership from the United States. Canadian-based companies hoping to become active in the U.S. health industry are seeking not just markets and partnerships with American corporations, but also experience they can carry back across the border to reshape what they view as Canada's outdated, anachronistic, and – worst of all – nonprofit health-care system. But corporate perceptions of the U.S. health-care system are in sharp contrast to individual Canadians' view of it as a looming and frightening spectre. In fact, the last thing Canadians want for the domestic health sector is the profit-driven, market-based U.S. system that has brought financial ruin, shorter life spans, and higher infant mortality rates to the American people.

Insuring the uninsured

The United States is host to large, aggressive, and competitive health corporations that claim their dominance of the market has created a system of the highest quality and efficiency in the world. Such claims are greeted with disbelief by the growing legions of American citizens who have little or no access to services because the price tag is too high. Access to the U.S. health system is denied to tens of millions of low- and middle-income Americans who do not qualify for public health-insurance programs, who are not covered by employer-sponsored health plans, who cannot afford the premiums charged by private insurers, or who are excluded from coverage because of chronic conditions such as asthma or diabetes. The result is that 72 percent of health-care services are consumed by only 10 percent of the population. The U.S. system of health care is in chaos, riddled with fraud and based on gross contradictions and distortions. It offers the best care for the fewest number of people, and this is its greatest accomplishment.[1]

The health-reform initiative of the early 1990s, when President Bill Clinton attempted to regulate competition in the insurance industry, precipitated a surge of corporate restructuring designed to undermine any move that would threaten profits earned in the health business. Canadian health-insurance companies, working hard to increase opportunities on the domestic front, were among those who shuddered at the thought of more government intervention in the U.S. health market. Six Canadian insurers were among the top twenty-five premium earners in a U.S. market comprised of some 1500 health-insurance companies. Manulife, Sun Life, Great West Life, CrownX, Canada Life, and North American Life watched with unease as Americans looked to their northern neighbour's single-payer plan for ideas about how to change their own profit-driven and chaotic system, known among Wall Street investors as the "sick business." As the U.S. and Canadian insurance industry prepared to join the most expensive lobby in the country's history to defeat Clinton's already watered-down proposal to bring "managed competition" to the health industry, Canadian life insurers and health companies must have felt an unwelcome tremor of déjà vu.

Health-care reform in the United States over the decade from the mid-1980s to the mid-1990s was situated almost entirely in the arena of funding cuts, a course followed by most governments in Canada during roughly the same period. In 1991, U.S. health-care expenditures reached $662 billion a year (12 percent of GDP) and were predicted – accurately, as events proved – to continue t their upward spiral. Public funds covered 40 percent of these costs through two programs established in the 1960s: Medicaid was paid for jointly by state and federal governments to provide coverage for the very poor; Medicare was a federal program for the elderly and disabled. The remaining 60 percent of health costs was financed by private payments that flowed either through insurers in the form of premiums or directly to companies to pay for services, drugs, and medical or other devices.

Yet despite such heavy spending, more than 33 million Americans lacked any protective health insurance whatsoever and millions more were inadequately covered. The fastest growing segment of the uninsured was American children, who made up one third of the total and whose parents could afford neither health insurance nor medical services. Low-income workers employed in small businesses, many of which were cancelling employee health benefits in the face of escalating premiums, also were joining the uninsured in alarming numbers. The situation for the American people has worsened since the health-reform initiatives of the Clinton administration went up in smoke in 1995; today, an estimated 45 million people lack any health insurance whatsoever, and the number who are inadequately covered continues to escalate. Children, women, the elderly, the disabled, blacks, and Latinos suffer disproportionately from lack of access to physicians and services. Seventy-five percent of the uninsured are employed or dependants of employed workers. In many ways, looking at the U.S. health system is, for Canadians, a horrifying reminder of the way things used to be in their own country. It also may be a sign of horrifying things to come.[2]

State governments, along with the White House, began drafting plans to address what was referred to as "the problem of the uninsured" – a problem unique to the United States among industrialized countries – in the late 1980s. Almost all of the plans, and there were many, focussed on expanding Medicaid to cover more of the poor and unemployed. Successive funding cuts to Medicaid had reduced the number of poor people eligible for assistance from 65 percent of those living below the poverty level in the mid-1970s to 47 percent by 1994.

Reform proposals for Medicare also came from the White House on a regular basis. Between 1987 and 1993 the percentage of large employers who provided health benefits to retirees shrank from 57 percent to only 35 percent. These abandoned retirees turned to Medicare for help, sparking calls for benefit reductions before the public program collapsed in bankruptcy.

The main victims of funding cuts were those who worked for small companies – along with their families – who did not qualify for either Medicaid or Medicare and could not afford private insurance premiums. Successive proposals from one government after another, designed to placate advocates of a single-payer system by extending health benefits to the uninsured, met with fierce resistance from the corporate sector.[3]

The powerful Health Insurance Association of America (HIAA), alarmed that politicians might come up with a scheme damaging to the industry's interests, jumped into the emerging debates armed with proposals of its own. In February 1990 the HIAA outlined a set of principles that it said would prevent health insurers from denying coverage to high-risk employers with fewer than twenty-five employees, even if a large number of employees had pre-existing conditions. Under the HIAA plan, benefit payments to high-risk workers could not be delayed beyond a one-year waiting period, and once workers were enrolled their coverage could not be cancelled because medical bills for an individual were high. Workers would not lose medical coverage if they switched jobs – an attractive selling point in a country where interrupted employment involves the loss of one's coveted health-insurance policy. The insurance industry claimed that its plan would guarantee coverage to 10 million American workers and their families, leaving the remaining uninsured to be covered by a beefed up Medicaid program.[4]

The insurance industry's many proposals during the 1980s and 1990s, however, were mainly designed to subvert any discussions that highlighted the benefits of a single-payer, universal, nonprofit, public insurance program. The industry also insisted on upholding practices that would enable it to shift costs from one group, such as big business, to less-powerful groups such as small employers and individual employees. Under the HIAA's proposed plan, for example, insurers would continue to vary premium prices by industry and by the age mix of a small company's workforce. Known as "cherry-picking," this practice enabled businesses with young, healthy, male workers and few industrial accidents to obtain health-insurance policies for relatively low premiums, while other, mainly smaller businesses paid rates up to eight times higher for fewer or more restricted benefits. During the 1980s, some smaller companies were subject to rate increases of up to 400 percent after employees were diagnosed with a high-cost disease such as cancer. Increases of this magnitude caused many employers to cancel benefits altogether, face bankruptcy, or either lay off or drop the employee in question from the health plan. In response the HIAA proposed to keep the lid on rate increases and to create a pool funded by insurers to cover high-risk subscribers, who would still pay a higher premium for coverage but within a narrower range of high and low rates.

The HIAA plan was a complicated and cumbersome proposal designed primarily to divert attention away from the American people's growing interest in Canada's government-run health-insurance system. It had the added benefit of creating new opportunities for insurers that could expand their markets with watered-down insurance policies more affordable to small employers. "With insurers willing to go a long way toward making [health insurance] more affordable," concluded *Fortune* magazine, "a government mandate now would be premature." But the HIAA's proposals were overtaken by another private-sector initiative, one that would increase the power and control of the insurance industry and threaten the existence of the nonprofit sector across the country.[5]

The birth of managed care

To say the health-insurance industry is reviled by the American public is an understatement, but this revulsion is in sharp contrast to the favoured treatment the industry has received from Congress and state regulators. Among major industries in the U.S., the insurance sector is the least regulated, generally free of laws governing price-fixing, monopoly control, anti-trust, market-share arrangements, or bundling (in which customers are forced to buy one kind of insurance they don't need in order to get the policy they do). The power and influence of the U.S. life- and health-insurance industry is matched only by the staggering worth of its consolidated assets, which in 1994 reached almost $2 trillion.

In the 1970s and 1980s a different kind of health-care delivery system began to emerge across the United States. Health maintenance organizations, or HMOs, were the creation of Henry Kaiser, a ship-building magnate, in 1942. The Kaiser HMO hired physicians, paid them a salary or capitation fees, and went beyond the typical employer-sponsored health-insurance plan. Kaiser's HMO not only offered prepaid medical insurance for Kaiser employees, but provided medical services as well, delivered in company-owned hospitals or community clinics. After World War II the company expanded its nonprofit HMO throughout the state of California, giving residents a welcome alternative to the insurance industry.

In 1973 President Richard Nixon's administration enacted the HMO Act, which required employers with twenty-five or more employees to provide prepaid health insurance through health maintenance organizations. The Act was Nixon's response to rumblings across the country for a Canadian-style single-payer health-insurance system. The HMO strategy, said Paul Ellwood, a Nixon consultant whose idea it was, "offers a common cause for the collaboration of the professional, public and private enterprise sectors of the health industry ... [and is] a feasible alternative to a nationalized health system." The HMO Act, coupled with the increased use of technology and medical specialists, changed the status of primary care physicians (or general practitioners) in the health system. By 1981, three out of five primary care physicians were on salary, many of them in HMOs, and another 25 percent worked under contract with hospitals. A decade later, the average income of a general practitioner was US$93,000, compared to $200,000 for specialists.

Not surprisingly, only one quarter of new doctors were entering primary care in the United States in the decades following the HMO Act. The emphasis in the "sick business" was, naturally enough, on illness, an emphasis that has increased the power of specialists – the "pros" who intervene at a moment of trauma and crisis – and decreased the role of primary care doctors who work with patients at a level of prevention. Specialists operated outside the salaried HMO system, but often worked in a group practice under contract to HMOs and, increasingly, private insurers. Group practices became popular among physicians who wanted to be part of a "marketing group" to cut down on the amount of resources required for billing and collection, an aspect of the business that often took up to 40 percent of a physician's revenues.[6]

When HMOs spread through the American landscape, they were seen as an alternative to the limited options offered by insurers and often were described as the "counterculture" of health care in the U.S. Most of the original HMOs were nonprofit physician group practices that offered integrated health services in community-based medical facilities. Patients covered by an HMO insurance policy could walk into a clinic run by the HMO for eye exams, blood tests, physical examinations, physiotherapy sessions, or consultations – one-stop shopping that was more convenient than travelling from one provider to another. Many nonprofit HMOs encouraged community input into how the facility operated to ensure the services they provided, and the hours they were open, met the needs of their clientele. The administrative overhead was substantially lower than that of commercial insurers, doctors' offices, and hospitals, though it was still substantially higher than that of Canada's government-run plans. By the 1990s, when insurance companies cast their eyes on HMOs as potential acquisitions, they saw an organizational structure, including the integrated approach to health care, that was a market-tested vehicle through which for-profit managed care could be delivered.

The first primitive step towards managed care in the United States was probably taken by Ronald Reagan, a stalwart supporter of the insurance industry. In a major effort to control Medicare and Medicaid payments to hospitals, Reagan won Congressional support in the early 1980s for "inpatient prospective payment," or Diagnostic Related Groupings (DRGs). Under the legislation, the government drew up a list of diagnoses and the way each one should be treated. These diagnostic and therapeutic procedures, including appropriate length of hospital stays, were then tied to a predetermined payment schedule. It was the strongest regulatory legislation since the enactment of Medicare and Medicaid in 1965, and while it succeeded in curbing hospitals that "milked Medicare" by keeping patients in beds for as long as possible, it also resulted in "DRG patients" being discharged before they were ready. The legislation also failed to attain the objectives laid out by the Reagan administration. Two years after DRGs were introduced, hospitals recorded their highest profits ever, and government officials expressed concern that hospitals were fraudulently billing the government by submitting claims for "high paying DRGs" when a lower cost procedure would have sufficed.[7]

Large corporations, alarmed at the rising cost of hospital and physician services during the decade, responded by tightening up their own internal control measures such as second opinions, peer and preadmission reviews, and prepaid group plans. They pressed insurance companies to implement cost-saving measures, which the companies did – by shifting the cost of insurance from big employers to small, denying coverage to high-risk groups and people with pre-existing conditions, and charging employees higher deductibles. The result was that large employers and insurers were able to download the costs of insurance to individuals and small businesses, even as overall health costs and the number of uninsured rose.[8]

The first formal managed care arrangement was introduced in March 1988 at the Allied Signal Corporation in New Jersey, an auto parts, aerospace, and chemical company with health-care costs rising by 39 percent a year. Allied Signal's goal was to set up a three-year contract with an insurer who could hold premium rate increases to a minimum. In exchange the insurer would net $1 billion to provide coverage to the company's 50,000 employees. The winning bid on the contract was from the Cigna Corporation, which promised to keep cost increases in the single digits in each of the three contract years. The formula to pare down medical costs required a reversal in corporate America's thinking. Whereas most industries derived their success – and profits – from increased productivity and output, the secret of managed care's success was less, not more, service delivery. By 1991, the idea had caught fire in boardrooms across the country. Meanwhile, back at

Allied Signal, employees bitterly complained about the loss of long-standing health benefits and the refusal of Cigna to pay for visits to doctors not on the insurer's roster.[9]

The growing concern in the United States about rising health-care costs pushed insurance companies, the target of increasing critical attention from employers whose business and premiums they sought, to divert attention away from their handsome profit margins and towards cost control. Indulging in an unusual round of self-criticism for allowing hospitals and doctors to overtreat, overprescribe and overbill, insurers vowed to manage health care in a more socially responsible manner. After all, insurers said, they were paying for much of the health care delivered to millions of customers, whose premiums were increasing by 15 to 20 percent a year because of wasteful spending practices, patient overuse of the health system, expensive technology, and unnecessary medical treatments.

Late in 1991, President George Bush, preparing for a national election, proposed a ten-year, $100 billion plan to achieve affordable "universal" coverage. This was in response to a new generation of Americans interested in Canada's single-payer system. At the heart of Bush's plan was a health-insurance card for "every American patient," issued by either a private or government plan. The whole scheme relied on a computerized health-care record "so that patients don't have to remember and don't have to repeat their medical history as they move through the system from primary care physician to specialists." To enable individuals to purchase private insurance cards, the White House promised a tax credit and subsidies for the working poor. Democratic senators in Congress called the plan "a gift of billions" to the insurance companies, labelling it the "Health Insurance Company Protection Act." But while commentators puzzled over how exactly cards and computers would achieve universal coverage, the HIAA praised the "vision ... that by the end of the decade every American will have a card."[10]

The response to Bush's card idea was mixed. "The insurance industry is not for the status quo," Peter Libassi of Travellers Insurance assured the American people in June 1992, six months after Bush launched his health reform crusade. "The current political situation is extremely dangerous to the insurance industry," he added, undoubt-edly thinking of the thirty-seven health reform proposals before Con-gress. But of greater concern to insurers and employers was a proposal known as "play-or-pay" that was being floated by the Bush White House in 1992. Play-or-pay would have required employers to buy health insurance for their workers ("play") or contribute a percentage of payroll to a government-created pool providing coverage ("pay").

Play-or-pay sent a wave of hysteria through the business commu-nity. Many small business owners threatened to shut their doors if they were forced to provide coverage for their employees, while the insurance industry declared that "play-or-pay" was a back door route to the dreaded Canadian-style single-payer system. Play-or-pay, fret-ted insurance industry executives, would overburden small busi-nesses unless payments for pool coverage were set low. But if payments were low, that would make the pool option more attractive for employ-ers than ever-rising insurance premiums. The pool would grow and private insurance would shrink, the industry logically concluded, while play-or-pay reforms would also lead to "burdensome regula-tion" of private health insurance.[11]

While the insurance industry generally praised Bush's "visionary" card idea, and blasted proposed legislation in Congress tabled by the Democratic party for a single-payer system, others worried that the Republicans were missing the boat. Boston-based Liberty Mutual, the world's largest provider of workers' compensation (and parent of Lib-erty Health), criticized the president for "chickening out on the real cost control issues." A year earlier Liberty vice president, Robert Laszewski, had proposed new insurance rules that would "transform insurers into watchdogs over medical expenditures" and "drive insur-ance companies to compete on the basis of which can best manage their customers' health care dollars." Accusing advocates of a single-payer system of searching for a "magic bullet," Laszewski echoed the words of OMA president Dr. W. K. Colbeck half a century earlier: "The real issue here ... is entirely over whether it's private sector insurance or government sector insurance." Either the insurance industry would manage care, he suggested, or the government would manage health insurance.[12]

The failure of Clinton's health-care reform

George Bush lost the election of 1992, and his health-reform efforts — feeble by any standard — went with him. Bill Clinton entered the White House on a platform that included a program that would be phased in to provide affordable "universal access to basic medical coverage" and a promise to "crack down on drug manufacturers and insurance companies." Clinton the candidate and Clinton the president, however, proved to be two very different people. During the election the candidate had deplored the denial of coverage to people with pre-existing conditions and the high infant mortality rates in the country. "Almost 60 million Americans have inadequate insurance, or none at all," he said, and he vowed to introduce radical reform measures to bring health care to every citizen.

In the minds of a growing number of Americans, any meaningful reform would have to include an expanded role for government and a significantly reduced one for private insurers. The average share of private insurance premiums paid by workers covered by employer-sponsored plans was $160 a month for individuals and $360 a month for a family of four in 1993. Under a government-sponsored, single-payer option proposed (but defeated) in California in 1994, employees who earned $35,000 a year would have paid $73 a month for "all medical care determined to be medically appropriate by the patient's health care provider." The math was not lost on working people.

But many employers — whose share of premiums ran between 50 percent and 80 percent — were also calculating the costs of private health benefits. Large corporations in particular, which competed with multinationals based outside the United States, grumbled about the advantages government-run health care gave to their competitors. In 1988 the Chrysler Corporation estimated that employee health benefits cost $700 for every car manufactured in the U.S., compared to only $223 for cars made in single-payer Canada. More to the point, Japanese automakers spent only $246 per car in their home country on health benefits, a significant cost advantage over their American competitors.[13]

The cost of private health insurance was driving a wedge between multinational employers and the insurance industry. Along with Lee Iacocca, head of Chrysler, others among the Fortune 500 were expressing interest in a Canadian-style system that would cost them less and offer more health services. "I never thought I would be in favour of a government health policy," said Robert Mercer, former chair of Goodyear Tire and Rubber, in late 1989, "but there are things that government must do. We have to spread the burden [of health-care costs]." With sentiments like these being publicly expressed by allies in the corporate community, the insurance industry pushed forward the idea of managed care. Insurance company executives promised that managed care would be the cornerstone – indeed, the last best hope – for U.S. health care in the future. "We're very committed to being a leading managed care company," James McLane of Aetna promised, "[and] that's where we're applying our resources."

The entrenchment of managed care coincided with Clinton's health-reform initiatives during 1993-1994 and was the response of an insurance industry feeling the pent-up hostility from a broad spectrum of American society. In its basic form, managed care divided the health industry into buyers (insurers and employers) and sellers (hospitals, doctors and other health-care providers). By banding together, buyers could exert greater control over providers – what services they offered and to whom, how much they charged, and even the clinical procedures and practices used to nurse sick patients back to health. In theory, managed care would contain costs by disciplining providers while safeguarding the interests of vulnerable patients and ensuring high-quality care. In practice, however, managed care meant an escalation of mergers and acquisitions – the insurance industry's method of banding together – and an erosion in both the amount and quality of care and of patients' rights, a deterioration of working conditions for all health-care workers (including primary care physicians), and an alarming reduction in the number of qualified health-care professionals. In many cases, managed care was a life-threatening solution to the U.S. medical crisis.

To support its move to managed care, the insurance industry relied heavily on the use of so-called medically based protocols that roughly emulated the DRGs of the Reagan era. In 1990 a Seattle-based consulting firm called Milliman & Robertson, Inc., published a guidebook of protocols to "help cost-conscious insurers say no." It was the perfect accessory for insurance executives who knew nothing about medicine but everything about how to make money. Called "the Supreme Court of medical insurance," Milliman & Robertson increased sales of its guidebook from an original run of 300 to more than 6000 by 1995. The books also provided administrative and clinical advice to many doctors and nurses who acted as consultants to some of the largest insurance corporations in the United States. Written by former insurance industry executive Richard L. Doyle, the guidelines now run to six volumes covering hospital admissions and stays, doctors' office treatments, home health care, dentistry, drug prescriptions, and rehabilitation aimed at getting injured workers back to work as soon as possible.

Critics of the guidebooks charged that Milliman & Robertson consulted with its growing clientele of insurers, foregoing the expert advice of medical societies and physician colleges to develop the guidelines. However, the idea of standardizing medical treatment struck a chord with employers and insurers alike. Many employers had championed the introduction of Total Quality Management and other industrial reengineering schemes during the 1980s. Such protocols – where workers were heavily supervised by quality control managers who carefully monitored how each screw was turned – had worked (at least for employers) in the auto industry, so it was an easy step for employers to believe they could work in the health industry, too.

The Milliman & Robertson guidelines placed a heavy emphasis on "refusals and delays [for surgery] unless a patient's state is serious and painful and other treatments have failed," while treatments by specialists for those with chronic diseases such as epilepsy or diabetes were denied in favour of lower-cost general practitioners. The company said that if its standards were strictly implemented, health plans could cut the length of hospital stays by two thirds, while saving "at least" 15 percent in medical insurance billings. Of course Milliman and Roberts also promised that quality care and the patient's well being would benefit by the increased attention given their treatment by insurance case managers.[14]

Armed with such seemingly scientific prescriptions for standards of care and treatment, insurers were more than ready when Bill Clinton outlined his plans to provide universal health insurance for Americans in September 1993. While a majority of Americans polled said they preferred a single-payer system, the Health Securities Act proposed by the president fell far short of these demands. Instead, Clinton's plan would enable the government to regulate – or manage – competition through 100 quasi-public state and regional health alliances across the country. Each alliance would act as a purchasing cooperative, negotiating rates and fees with hospitals, physicians, and other providers. The alliances also would negotiate with large insurance companies and HMOs (almost all of which were now controlled by the ten largest insurers) to provide individuals within their region a choice from among three different health plans. Each plan would offer the minimum benefits required by the federal government, although insurers would set their own premiums in the negotiating process with each alliance.

The legislation banned discrimination based on age, sex, health status, or medical costs and required employers to insure all of their employees, paying 80 percent of the premium cost charged by the alliance. Workers could purchase additional coverage or, through collective bargaining or other arrangements, obtain additional coverage from their employers. The almost 46 million people whose incomes were less than 150 percent of the poverty line and who passed a means test would be eligible for a subsidy to purchase private insurance, while Medicare would be refocussed to provide coverage to the still-uninsured. Small businesses – which also would be means-tested – could obtain subsidies to limit their premiums to a fixed percentage of payroll. Health plans with more than 5000 participants were exempted from the health alliances, thus legislating a separate tier for large employers and insurance corporations that could make their own arrangements.[15]

The Clinton bill's prime focus on cost containment and managed competition mirrored the theories of the Jackson Hole group, a think tank of big-business executives and conservative academics headed by Paul Ellwood. Ellwood was widely respected for his success in averting a move to Canadian-style health care during the 1970s with the introduction of Nixon's HMO Act. The think tank was financed generously by the insurance and pharmaceutical industries, large employers, and professional associations to advance theories such as the market-driven managed competition idea. It played an important role in developing the Clinton plan, with its underlying assumption that the U.S. health-care crisis stemmed from a lack of competition rather than from the presence of the private health-insurance industry.[16]

The Jackson Hole group, while generally supporting the Clinton proposal, was disappointed with elements of the plan, which it said could be "a giant step toward a single-payer system," especially if the health industry failed to turn public opinion around. However, with the key elements of managed competition woven into the proposal thanks to the group's significant input, there was still hope that "every part of the ... plan can be modified in a satisfactory way. All the pieces are there. We're just talking about how you tweak it to make it work."[17]

But the Clinton proposal needed more than a "tweak" to overcome the mounting opposition from every corner of the political spectrum. On the business side, the most vociferous opponents gathered under the umbrellas of the Health Insurance Association of America, the Chambers of Commerce, and the National Federation of Independent Business – all representing small business and small to medium-sized insurers. Large insurance corporations and employers came together in the Coalition for Managed Competition, which was organized to lobby for the "tweaks" referred to by the Jackson Hole group. Not surprisingly, the coalition's proposals would do even more to protect insurers and corporate health-care providers while shifting costs to small business and individuals.

Big business was generally supportive of the plan's mandated employer contributions (or "employer mandates"), universal coverage, and a continuation of the employer-based system of insurance, but opposed "price controls and bureaucrats," taxed benefits, and regulations that would cap premiums. Although large insurers would have been among the major beneficiaries of the Clinton plan, they nonetheless strongly opposed the increased regulation of the industry by the federal government. There was strong support for universal coverage – as long as it was provided by private insurers – a move that would end the indirect subsidy that was included in hospital charges to insured patients for the uninsured whose admission to hospital was typically through the emergency department. The Coalition for Managed Competition maintained a posture of lukewarm support while spending huge sums to expose the flaws of the system in Canada and in other countries where health insurers played a negligible role. By early 1994, however, the Business Roundtable and top executives in the Fortune 500, won over by the managed care revolution, announced they were withdrawing support for the Clinton plan. Their main concern, they said, was cost control, and the insurance industry's managed care idea was a perfect, free-enterprise fit.

The hospital sector, whose members worried that cuts to Medicare and Medicaid would seriously undermine quality care (and a lucrative source of revenue), pushed for hospital-run HMOs as the prime insurers in the new system. Physicians, who had an influential voice in the debate, were split between those who opposed government regulation, Medicare benefit reductions, and spending caps, and a growing number who were actively supporting the single-payer option.[18]

Small and medium-sized insurance companies, united in the HIAA, were among the most vociferous opponents of health-care reform. If Clinton's plan were implemented, they said, they quite simply would not survive, unlike the largest insurers, which would expand their control of the industry. (Many astute observers concluded that this was, in fact, the intention.) Health insurers, large and small, spent $25 million on political donations to encourage sympathetic members of Congress to work hard against any proposals that would damage the industry, while the HIAA spent another $20 million to defeat the single-payer model. Small business mounted a ferocious assault on the Clinton plan, warning of major job losses if employer-mandated coverage was implemented. Small business and the HIAA worked overtime to defeat Clinton's plan and – with an election coming at the end of 1996 – Clinton as well.[19]

News coverage of the single-payer option was sparse during debates on the Clinton reform proposal, despite strong support across the country and more than 100 Congressional sponsors of a bill that would have made it a reality. The most popular news program in the country, ABC's *World News Tonight*, referred to the single-payer option once during all of 1993. On April 1 of that year, when President Clinton was presented with a petition supporting a single-payer system that was signed by over a million people, not one major media outlet covered the event. City council members in Buffalo, New York, a short drive from the Canada-U.S. border, took turns staging a one-day fast to support the city's demands for a single-payer system similar to their northern neighbour's in August 1994. This was another important event that received no coverage.[20]

By the middle of 1994, more than $100 million had been spent in a full-tilt campaign to defeat both the Clinton plan and the growing movement for a single-payer system. Newspaper editorials and columnists across the country (especially those in the *New York Times*, four of whose twelve directors sat on the boards of insurance companies) defended the record of private enterprise, asserting that it alone was responsible for a U.S. health-care system envied the world over for its innovation and bold technological advances. The efforts of this campaign were aided and abetted by several Canadian luminaries such as Michael Walker of the Vancouver-based Fraser Institute. While admitting that Canada spent much less on health than the U.S., Walker said this fact had led many American lawmakers to conclude erroneously "that rapidly rising U.S. health care costs indicate that free markets are an inferior way of delivering health care." Not so, he said, asking "Why is it desirable to spend a low fraction of Canadian GNP on health care?" – a condition that was detrimental to the profit margins of private insurers and corporate providers.[21]

In the meagre coverage of the single-payer plan advocated by unions and consumer groups, there was no shortage of outright lies in the attack on Canada's universal medicare system. The *New York Times* maintained that Canadian women, for example, had to wait months for a simple Pap smear, a charge vehemently denied by Canada's ambassador to the United States two weeks later. One assertion, repeated endlessly in newspapers and television broadcasts, was that Canadian patients could not choose their own physicians. Americans were warned that socialized medicine denied basic human rights, in particular the sacred right to jump to the head of the queue if one had the requisite cash and class privilege. The irony of such charges, given that managed care was based on a denial of physician choice, was lost on, or denied by, most business and insurance industry leaders.

But if business seemed less than solid in its response to the health-reform bill, divided between large and small interests, the movement for a single-payer system was all but undone by the proposed legislation. Hostility and mistrust towards the insurance industry was high, with polls showing that 90 percent of Americans consistently expressed strong dissatisfaction with the way the health system worked (or didn't) and 62 percent expressing a preference for Canada's single-payer plan. With such strong support for a fundamental change in the U.S. system, what prevented advocates of the Canadian option from mobilizing the American people and winning their goal?

Many single-payer proponents feared that if they failed to rally behind the Clinton plan, Americans would be left with the same problems that had given rise to demands for change in the first place. However, these proponents criticized the health-reform bill for failing to address what they viewed as the single most flawed characteristic of the U.S. system: the role of private insurance companies. In fact, critics argued, Clinton's plan would increase the largest and most powerful insurers' control over the health-care system by defeating any attempts to lower costs and establish universal coverage. Clinton's proposal would simply open the public purse to pay higher premium rates for high-risk patients historically excluded by insurers. "Insurance executives could recommend batteries of unproven screening tests for all enrollees, dubiously labelling millions with premium-inflating diagnoses like 'borderline diabetes' or 'early Alzheimers' ... What the Clinton plan would do is enrich the biggest insurers and wipe out small insurers and individual medical practices."[22]

Many other groups, in particular those representing seniors, supported the bill's generous benefits package, especially coverage provided for long-term care, home care, and nursing care. Unions, involved in a very public campaign against the North American Free Trade Agreement and Clinton's support for NAFTA, appeared reluctant to throw another round of darts at the president on his health-care reform initiative, especially given the right-wing assault on the plan. While the Oil, Chemical and Atomic Workers union and the United Electrical Workers supported a Congressional bill on the single-payer plan introduced early in 1994, most unions endorsed the Clinton proposal. The American Federation of Labour-Congress of Industrial Organizations (AFL-CIO), whose support for single-payer had been lukewarm, joined with many big-business groups calling for employer mandates and opposing premium caps, cost containment rules, and taxed health benefits. Meanwhile, a broad array of groups including Physicians for a National Health Plan, Ralph Nader's Public Citizen, the Grey Panthers, and Americans for Democratic Action worried that the trade union movement's support for the Clinton proposal was "foreclosing the single payer option."[23]

In the end, Clinton's only success in his ill-fated efforts to reform health care was the fragmentation of support for meaningful, funda-mental change in the United States. As the debates about health-care reform dragged on through 1994, the American public became more and more confused. In addition to Clinton's proposal, Congress seemed to be drowning in health-care legislative initiatives, all purportedly aimed at extending coverage to the uninsured, which by this time had increased in number to 40 million people, most of them children and workers employed in the "high-risk" small-business sector. The only bill that seemed to come close to what the American people wanted called for a single-payer system and was introduced by Congressmen John McDermott and Paul Wellstone. By the fall, Congress was com-pletely immobilized, with support for any single initiative fragmented and divided. An election campaign was on the horizon and quiet retreat now seemed the best plan of all.

The market takes control

With public policymakers in total disarray and a White House strat-egy of abandonment in full swing, the corporate sector breathed a sigh of relief and moved swiftly to implement its own reform plan. This effort took two forms, neither of which had anything to do with extending insurance to the uninsured. The first was a corralling of large numbers of patients into HMOs with a managed care ethos that promised lower costs and increased efficiency in return for limits on patient care. The second was a rapid consolidation among insurers, providers, and pharmaceutical corporations, and an aggressive acquisition of nonprofit HMOs by large insurance companies. "The system is finally correcting itself," said David Colby of Columbia/HCA, the largest health corporation in the world, while Art Young, benefits manager at Hewlett-Packard enthused, "Where we have a competitive market, it's really working."[24]

The growth of managed care was in large part the result of a war waged by insurance companies to seize control of the health-care system from physicians, who acted as gatekeepers – overpaid gatekeepers as far as insurers were concerned. If patients were responsible for a profligate overuse of services (and thus for high overall U.S. expenditures), they were ably assisted, in the insurance companies' view, by greedy doctors who benefitted from the fee-for-service method of payment. In addition, doctors were in a direct conflict of interest since they, not the insurer, prescribed the services for which they were generously paid. In order to reshape health-care delivery and address the concerns of employers who bought their policies, insurers began herding patients from indemnity plans to managed care HMOs.

By mid-1997, more than 75 percent of all HMOs in the United States were operating as for-profit managed care companies, up from 18 percent in the early 1980s. Almost all of the HMOs in the for-profit industry had been transformed from not-for-profit alternative providers of health insurance and services through conversions, mergers, or buyouts. Blue Cross – long a symbol of nonprofit service – was also converting to for-profit status, and in 1996 the national organization revoked its longstanding rule that any provider bearing the Blue Cross name must operate as a nonprofit company. The cost of all these conversions and buyouts was almost $20 billion, while salaries, stock options, and bonuses for executives in the new companies reached into the millions of dollars. The price of the new managed care miracle was high – and someone was going to have to pay. That "someone" was, inevitably, patients, who saw sharp increases in deductibles and co-payments for services. A study published in a U.S. health journal in 1997 reported that hospital co-payment fees for managed care patients had risen by over 450 percent between 1987 and 1993, while patients' share of doctors' fees had tripled.[25]

Many nonprofit HMOs formed for-profit joint ventures with the corporate sector in order to retain their charitable tax status while tapping new sources of revenue. In 1996 many states began requiring HMOs converting to for-profit status to form charitable foundations to fund indigent care in their communities. But foundations, argued Donald Stewart, president of Kansas Health Foundation, were "moving toward a much broader, non-illness-oriented definition of health" and should not be required to fund health care for the poor. In addition, such activities did not adequately raise the profile of the parent corporation – which preferred allocating funds to the arts, Little League teams, or other nonhealth activities that provided a lucrative tax write-off. "For-profitization will make the problem of the uninsured more vivid," said Martin Schroeder, president of another health-care foundation. "It will be harder and harder for people who don't have health insurance to get care."[26]

Altogether, some 164 million insured Americans were covered by managed care companies in 1997, many of them HMOs owned by the largest insurers, and physicians and hospitals were on radically altered payment schemes. Instead of fee-for-service, doctors were placed on capitation and paid a flat monthly rate for each patient on their roster, regardless of the patient's health status. Similarly, hospitals were paid a fixed price for each case in accordance with each HMO's schedule, many of them based on Milliman and Roberts' "how to say no" guidelines. Fixed capitation and case rates turned sick patients into money-losers, while the young and healthy who needed little or no medical attention were money-generators. HMO profits, as a result, were up, while coverage for those with pre-existing conditions, for children, for minority Americans, and for others deemed to be poor risks was down.[27]

The aggressive takeover of nonprofit HMOs by commercial insurers provoked a backlash among consumer groups who saw their benefits decreasing and control over their health care slipping into the hands of benefits managers and utilization consultants. "The new age of managed care has been ushered in with a lot of talk about consumer choice," said *Consumer Reports* magazine, a leading critic of the insurance industry. "It's an appealing picture, but today, it's a mirage." Instead, activists complained, employers offered restricted choices to their workers while information about services available on managed care plans was "limited and often misleading." In a large survey undertaken by *Consumer Reports*, "patients tended to be most satisfied with the not-for-profit plans, which still cling to a sense of mission that goes beyond the bottom line."[28]

By the end of 1997, the takeover of nonprofit health-care organizations by for-profit companies – activity that was almost entirely unregulated, unobserved, and undebated – represented the largest transfer of charitable assets in U.S. history. The corporate assault on the nonprofit sector led U.S. health-care activists and consumer groups to campaign for restrictions on the sale and transfer of assets to for-profit corporations. When fifteen Blue Cross/Blue Shield groups restructured into for-profit managed care companies, activists in several states lobbied for legislation against such transfers of charity assets. Groups argued that the assets of the nonprofit "Blues" – which totalled as much as $60 billion in 1996 – had been acquired "because consumers and taxpayers bankrolled [the companies]" and had given them "tax exemptions, periodic infusions of capital ... and, in one instance, discounts on charges at hospitals." California activists succeeded in forcing Blue Cross to shift $3.2 billion to two nonprofit charities after the company converted to for-profit status. In Colorado, legislation was passed that required nonprofit insurers and providers converting to "corporate managed care profit centres," as they were cheerily described, to obtain a fair assessment of the market value of their assets and to transfer those assets to a philanthropic foundation. Columbia/HCA's bid to take over Ohio Blue Cross was rejected by state regulators in early 1997 after questions arose about the valuation of the nonprofit insurer and about Columbia's plan to pay $19 million in consulting fees to the top Blue Cross officials who negotiated the deal.[29]

Consumer complaints were rooted in the shift of control over health care from individuals to insurers and employers. Under traditional indemnity insurance, patients were able to choose their doctors, who then coordinated the care they required, including specialists and drug and rehabilitative therapy. Under managed care, insurers gave employers a list of doctors and services covered by the plan. Individuals had to choose a doctor from the list, and the doctor coordinated care from among the limited services on the insurer's list. The insurance contract was subject to change every year and so, therefore, was the list of doctors, drugs, and services patients had access to. Critics argued such practices interfered with the long-term relationship between patients and their doctors and enforced a lack of continuity that undermined preventive care. Defenders of the new system claimed patients had to make some compromises to keep premiums in check and to discourage the overuse of health-care services. New studies, many of them by groups such as Jackson Hole, Ernst and Young, and Price Waterhouse, supported insurance company claims that the "quality" of services under managed care was the same or better than before, despite public perceptions to the contrary.[30]

Managed care plans also came under fire for offering incentives and bonuses to physicians who denied care to their patients, thereby saving insurers and employers money. While Canadian doctors, led by the CMA, were debating the merits of private insurance to help finance health care, their U.S. colleagues were moving towards open rebellion against insurers obsessed with increasing profit margins at the expense of high standards and quality care. Doctors complained about restrictions on the treatment options they could recommend to their patients and on the necessary tests and procedures they were able to perform. These criticisms reached a fever pitch at the end of 1996, forcing Washington to limit HMO bonuses paid to doctors as a reward for denying services to Medicare and Medicaid patients. At the same time, Congress began a debate about whether and how it should manage managed care, a move denounced by the insurance industry. Liberty Mutual's suggestion that "either the government would manage health insurance — or the insurance industry would manage care," was back on the agenda.[31]

Physicians, meanwhile, viewing their new status as members of the working class with dismay, began organizing in earnest. Over 45 percent of doctors were now on salary at managed care companies, hospitals, and government agencies, and they found their employers were able to dictate salary levels and dismiss them without cause. Their conditions of employment, including treatment practices and "gag" rules that prevented their discussing the full range of options with their patients, were set entirely by the employer. Unionization looked like a practical way to regain some control over working conditions and to reestablish professional autonomy. Unions such as the First National Guild for Health Care Providers of the Lower Extremities (representing podiatrists), the Federation of Physicians and Dentists, and the Union of American Physicians and Dentists saw their membership more than double as doctors reacted angrily to managed care. "This isn't about money or power," said one Florida physician. It was about "getting managed care off [our] backs when it comes to making decisions about the care that patients get and when they get it."[32]

But the struggle *was* about money and power. In 1995 the cost of HMO coverage dropped for the first time in ten years by 3.9 percent, largely due to a drop or delay in the number of tests and procedures, decreased referrals to specialists, fewer hospital admissions and shorter stays, and "reined-in" benefits. The new rules were necessary, claimed experts such as Milliman and Roberts (who also wrote them), because half of "unnecessary" hospital days were due to doctors' failure to send patients home early. Doctors employed by or on contract with for-profit managed care HMOs were required to adhere to "medical cookbooks" prescribing outpatient surgery for mastectomy patients, two days in hospital for caesarean deliveries, and three days for heart transplant and bypass patients. Employers embarking on America's annual ritual of renewing or changing their health coverage began using such guidelines to assess the dollar value of their managed care plans, often forcing employees into an endless search for new "listed" doctors when another plan was adopted. Health care, claimed a battery of consultants, was a business "no different from any other," patients were "money-generating biological structures," and, best of all, HMOs were earning "extraordinary profits ... and using that money to expand in other parts of the country."[33]

At the end of 1996, newspapers in both Canada and the United

States trumpeted the success of managed care, comparing the failure of U.S. attempts to reform the health-care system in a public policy forum with the more efficient, streamlined process of the marketplace. Unlike the "ponderous decision-making" in Congress, the private sector had finally kicked a dent in the fee-for-service model, the charging structure mainly responsible for insulating doctors and patients from the true costs of health care – costs known only to insurance companies and employers who paid the bills. The proof of this formula lay in the fact that as health expenditures as a percentage of GDP held steady at just under 14 percent, the fee-for-service model was on the decline. That rickety and old-fashioned standard had been replaced by managed care, which transferred "the responsibility – or risk – for the provision of individuals' health care" to large, corporate buyers and sellers. "The marketplace is transforming itself," one commentator chirped, "and is delivering health care at reduced costs or at a slower rate of price increase." Predictions of further declines were beamed optimistically across the U.S. and Canada, while consolidation in the sector was "set to continue."[34]

The replacement of fee-for-service with salaries and capitation in the medical profession was historically a goal of progressive reformers to minimize costs and protect patients from unethical or unscrupulous abuse by physicians. Insurers were quick to point to their success in eliminating fee-for-service in managed care plans. But DRG-type fee schedules were alive and well and prospering in the U.S. health-insurance industry. In 1996, for example, Liberty Mutual boasted it had saved $106 million in occupational medical costs in Florida due to "the use of the medical fee schedule" and "aggressive treatment and rehabilitation protocols" published in guidebooks prepared by actuaries such as Milliman and Roberts to minimize benefit payouts for patient care.[35]

Insurers complained of "thin profits" resulting from their attempts to hold down prices and increase enrollment during the health reform "scare," and pointed to a moderate 6.8 percent increase in assets from 1993 to 1994. But it was hard to feel much sympathy when "thin profits" meant an after-tax income of nearly US$12 billion, and a "moderate increase" equaled a US$122.04 billion rise in the value of insurers' assets, worth $2 trillion in 1994. The hundred top life and health insurers – which included Canadian companies – controlled fully 87 percent of the assets and profits in the insurance industry. The ten largest HMOs reported a combined $10.5 billion in liquid assets, otherwise known as pure cash. In the same year, premium income for health insurers totalled $300 billion, and a third of the premiums that went to HMOs were taken "off the top" in profit and administration fees.[36]

To increase their value among Wall Street investors, HMOs had to demonstrate a promising "medical-loss ratio" of benefits paid out compared to premiums coming in. The fewer benefits paid to patients, the higher the profit margins for the insurer and the more attractive the medical-loss ratio to investors. While the few remaining nonprofit HMOs spent roughly 90 percent of premium income on payments for their members' health care in the 1990s, for-profit companies registered medical-loss ratios of between 68 percent and 76 percent in 1994. The less an HMO spent on patient care, the better it would do on Wall Street.[37]

An increasing portion of these profits were derived from Medicare patients who were being encouraged by federal and state governments to join managed care HMOs in the hopes of saving money. These patients were being aggressively pursued by insurers because Medicare was a rich and regular payer. A marketer who delivered fifty signed-up Medicare patients a month to an HMO could earn as much as $190,000 a year, plus benefits. By early 1997, 5 million of Medicare's 38 million patients were enrolled in managed care HMOs. At the same time the General Accounting Office – the federal government's spending watchdog – reported that of $6 billion paid by Medicare to HMOs in California in 1995, $1 billion was in "excess payments" for inappropriate billings or services that were never delivered.

The promise of such rich rewards was overwhelming, and HMO insurers were locked in heated competition for the Medicare dollar. In August 1996, PacifiCare Health Systems Inc., a for-profit HMO in southern California, announced a $2.1 billion acquisition of fellow California giant, FHP International. The takeover created the fifth largest managed care company in the U.S. With more Medicare patients than any other managed care company – accounting for 25 percent of total enrollment, but 60 percent of the company's $3.7 billion in 1995 revenue – PacifiCare was well positioned to "dive deeper into the largely untapped and highly lucrative Medicare market."

The market was lucrative because the federal government allocated $26 billion in fees in 1997 to HMOs for disbursing payments to providers looking after Medicare enrollees. These costs were expected to increase to a stunning $141 billion by 2006 when an anticipated 14 million Medicare patients would be channelled into managed care HMOs.

PacifiCare and FHP had something in common besides their interest in Medicare patients. Both were under investigation by the federal government for allegedly overcharging for federal employees enrolled in their managed care plans. Nonetheless, Wall Street smiled on the deal. Shares were sent soaring on the stock market, while employees of the new company were warned to start thinking about alternative employment prospects.[38]

The potential for increased profits drove health and insurance companies to spin off, merge with, and acquire other health and insurance companies at a frenetic pace by the mid-1990s. In 1994, mergers and acquisitions in the U.S. health sector totalled $20 billion, up from $6 billion two years earlier. When added to the $22 billion in drug company deals, mergers in the health industry surpassed those of any other in the U.S. economy. "It's the corporatization of health care," said one Wall Street analyst. "And what's wrong with that?"

Unfortunately, as the *New York Times* soberly noted, "This restructuring has done nothing to ease the plight of the uninsured, whose numbers keep climbing." But, then, that was hardly the point. Revenues at the largest HMOs increased dramatically from millions to billions, and profit margins rose with them. Oxford Health Plan, for example, saw its revenues swell from $760 million in 1994 to $3.08 billion in 1996, largely the result of an acquisition binge begun four years earlier. The chaos and disruption in the U.S. health-care system as insurers and employers shifted to managed care resulted in a three-year, record-setting slowdown in overall cost increases, most of it extracted from the most vulnerable sections of the population. The number of uninsured continued to grow, with estimates reaching 45 million to 50 million in 1996. As many other Americans experienced service cuts and deteriorating benefits under managed care, CEOs at the largest health-care companies saw their already-rich compensation packages enriched even further.[39]

In early 1997, employers, actuaries, and health-industry analysts worried that managed care may have outlived its usefulness – health costs in the United States, they said, were poised to surge upwards again. In fact, costs already were surging for small businesses, some of whom had seen a 25 percent increase over the previous year. "We may have squeezed out all that we can through managed care," said a spokesperson for an employer coalition, while a medical cost tracker predicted "a return to double-digit health care inflation." The U.S. government saw its health premiums increase 8.5 percent in 1997, and private employers were not faring much better. Many managed care companies began seeking increases for 1998 of between 4 and 8 percent. "The HMOs have got to raise rates to keep Wall Street happy," said Lee Aurich of Kaiser Permanente, the California-based nonprofit HMO.[40]

The managed care revolution had reached its peak, and with unflagging determination Canadian insurers and health corporations were determined to bring the failed experiment to their own home turf.[41]

EIGHT

He Who Pays
the Piper ...

In 1991, Winnipeg's Seven Oaks General Hospital became one of the first large facilities in Canada to embrace the underlying principles of managed care when its CEO, Nick Kaplansky, implemented treatment guidelines that established how long patients needed to be hospitalized. The tough new guidelines, developed by a U.S. medical management company, were designed to send patients home earlier, Kaplansky said, so they could spend "more time ... recovering with their families." This was an improvement in the care Seven Oaks provided patients, he added, "because there's a better attitude and better support for them at home."

Businesses supporting Kaplansky's initiative claimed the hospital's rigid guidelines had a proven track record in the United States, where managed care HMOs were reducing hospital admissions and lowering insurance costs with the help of similar protocols. The dose of managed care dealt to Seven Oaks resulted in reduced hospital stays and the closure of 10 percent of its surgery beds, all of which, Kaplansky said, had saved $3 million. "If that's cookbook medicine," quipped *Canadian Business* magazine, "maybe it's time to ask for the recipe."[1]

But four years later, Kaplansky's recipe was used in ways the hospital had not foreseen. In January 1996 a committee looking at ways to reorganize the allocation of intensive care beds in Winnipeg's community hospitals recommended that all of the beds in Seven Oaks' intensive care unit (ICU) be closed – to save money. The bed closures, said the committee, would result in improved efficiencies and quality of service. Ignoring demographic trends that strongly suggested the need for acute-care beds in Winnipeg's community hospitals was on the rise, the reorganization committee said its goal was a reduction of patient days in hospital by 10 to 18 percent.

One Seven Oaks physician, Dr. Neil Lerner, charged that the committee was dominated by "medical empire builders" from the city's university teaching hospitals who used "unsubstantiated data, faulty statistics and arrogant and narrow-minded assumptions" to support its recommendations for a consolidation of ICU beds in the city. As patients, hospital staff, and physicians grappled with bed closures and empire builders in Winnipeg, the medicinal cookbook of competition and market rules was being promoted by adherents of private medicine, offering managed care solutions that were proven failures elsewhere on the continent.[2]

Fighting for the driver's seat

By the mid-1990s the business sector had launched a full attack on Canada's health-care system. Employers worried that the publicly funded system was inefficient, costly, and rationed through growing wait lists – and they turned increasingly to for-profit companies that promised to bring the managed care techniques employed in the U.S. to their Canadian operations. Actuaries gave the country "five years to fix health care" and joined with Vancouver's Fraser Institute to charge that the system faced a $1 trillion "unfunded liability." The only way to save medicare, they said, was to implement user fees, co-payments, and deductibles. It mattered not at all that the absence of direct cash payments was a key ingredient to Canada's universal health-care system. "Demographics and deficit pressures ... dictate that the days of unrestricted access to unlimited health care resources must soon end," the Canadian Institute of Actuaries warned.[3]

Undaunted by the upheaval and trauma associated with cuts in public health expenditures south of the border, Canadian business leaders – not a few of them representing U.S. subsidiaries – orchestrated an increasingly strident chorus about out-of-control public spending and growing deficits. A major focus of this concern was the one third, on average, of provincial budgets that went to health, creating what critics of medicare charged was an overwhelming fiscal crisis. With giant debt clocks ticking inexorably above their heads, Canadians learned that health-care spending, once a source of deep national pride, was now a major cause of the country's crippling debt – was, in fact, an international embarrassment. Not only did Canada spend more than any other nation on health care (with the exception, always bracketed, of the United States), but critics also claimed the system was a technological backwater characterized by long queues of patients waiting their turn at magnetic resonance imaging (MRI) machines and other scarce marvels of modern medicine. Waiting lists, said business-funded think tanks like the Fraser Institute, combined with restrictions on private-sector alternatives, were health-care rationing in disguise. Although the institute supported rationing access to services by imposing user fees, co-payments, and deductibles, it argued that middle-class Canadians with disposable incomes should be buying services from the private sector, something they were prevented from doing by the Canada Health Act. Reforms were urgently needed, according to the *Financial Post*, that addressed "the basic problem with medicare – the lack of purchasers."[4]

The Fraser Institute's complaints about waiting lists and the lack of private-sector alternatives were, at the very least, artful. In the mid-1980s the institute took part in a two-year federal government study of the structure and dynamics of the service sector and its component industries. A 1986 paper cowritten with the Institute for Research on Public Policy (IRPP) and entitled "Caring for Profit: Economic Dimensions of Canada's Health Industry" provided details of the rapid growth of the private health sector and of what was needed to support further expansion of the domestic industry. The paper established a framework for future discussions between health-care companies and the government about what the private sector required to increase profits in the delivery of health-care services, many of which were already being delivered by publicly funded, nonprofit providers.[5]

In addition, groups like the Fraser Institute had contributed handsomely to the fear and apprehension Canadians felt about the ability of governments to continue funding health services. In 1995, the group claimed, "there was a shortfall in current dollar terms of at least $1 trillion" in health-care funding. It was little wonder, therefore, "that governments are focused on reducing their expenditures." To control the deficit, the business institute said, "public sector costs should be reduced by creating incentives for those who can afford to do so to opt out of the public sector health care budget."[6]

The public, too, saw health-care cuts as a necessary if painful sacrifice to help governments wrestle the "deficit monster" to the ground, putting their shaken trust in the spirit and letter of the Canada Health Act to safeguard medicare. Health investors and their defenders, on the other hand, saw funding cuts as an "opportunity" to step into a growing gap in the provision of services: just as "B" follows "A," funding cuts and shortfalls meant increased waiting times, the removal of services from provincial health plans, the elimination of outpatient services from hospitals – and more health dollars diverted to the private sector. "There is clear empirical evidence," said the Fraser Institute, "that the introduction of market-based reforms benefits the health care sector." All one had to do, the think tank said, was look south of the border.[7]

Ironically, as the Fraser Institute attempted to rouse public demand for private-sector alternatives, U.S. state and federal governments were coming under increasing pressure to ban the cost-cutting solutions being implemented by managed care HMOs. "Drive-through" breast removals for cancer patients denied an overnight stay in hospital, denial of treatment options to insured patients, bonuses for doctors who denied care altogether, decisions about appropriate drug prescriptions made by actuaries, early hospital discharges, lack of patient choice in physicians – these were just a few of the qualities offered by the corporate health sector. Market medicine in the U.S. also succeeded in increasing infant mortality rates to the highest level among industrialized countries in 1994 – 9.1 per 1000 live births compared to

6.8 per 1000 births delivered in Canada's "government monopoly." Private-sector alternatives in the U.S. have also left the estimated 20 percent of the population who are uninsured in a deadly queue where entry to the health-care system is exclusively through the emergency ward of a charity hospital.[8]

Proponents of market medicine ignored these statistics and worked hard to present private-sector alternatives as the answer to growing wait lists and what they described as the poor performance of the publicly funded system. In 1996 the Fraser Institute published a study on waiting times for specialists across the country. The longest waits, the think tank said, were for elective treatment in three specialty areas: orthopedic surgery, cardiovascular surgery, and ophthalmology, the latter of which scored the worst record for waiting times. But the answer to lengthening queues was more complex than these private-sector proponents suggested and had more to do with adequate public funding and increased regulation of the medical profession, not the expansion of the for-profit health industry.

The Fraser Institute's study was based on the subjective observations offered by specialists who "in almost every instance" felt that waiting times were too long for treatment. "Waiting times for many operations and diagnostic tests," the institute said, "greatly exceed medically acceptable norms." In its 1996 study "Waiting Your Turn," the opinions of medical specialists with genuine concerns about their patients were used to support the Fraser Institute's contention that the "government's monopoly" was at the bottom of the problem. (Ironically, many of the same voices demanding "medically acceptable norms" to determine appropriate waiting times were also calling for definitions of "medical necessity" to determine what services could be excluded from public health plans.) "The private sector must become a larger part of the health care sector if Canada's health system is to be saved," the think tank advised nervous Canadians.[9]

But the Fraser Institute is not the only organization conducting studies of wait lists. In 1995 the Alberta branch of the Consumers' Association of Canada (CAC) investigated claims by private-health-care proponents that private clinics could offer faster service than the publicly funded hospital sector. In a survey of ophthalmology services at offices and clinics in five Alberta cities, the CAC asked how long a patient would have to wait for cataract surgery.

Three types of ophthalmologists were surveyed: those who operated only in the publicly funded hospital system; those who operated only in the private system; and those who operated in both. Patients whose doctors worked entirely in the private system waited between one day and four weeks for surgery, while those whose doctors worked only in the public system would wait an average of six weeks. But the waiting times for surgery in the public system were up to a year if the surgeon operated in both a hospital and private clinic. Patients whose doctors used both private and public operating rooms, the CAC's executive coordinator Wendy Armstrong concluded, would have the mistaken impression that the problem lay in the hospital, when in fact the problem was in the choice of physician. Long waiting times for ophthalmology, medicare supporters charged, had more to do with bumping "public pay" patients to the end of the queue in favour of higher-paying private payers.[10]

Wait lists in Canada are a frustrating experience for patients and their families, who sometimes must spend many long and anxious weeks waiting for an operation that will alleviate pain or enable an injured worker to return to his or her job. Physicians who juggle patients from public and private insurers are part of the problem, but an even more serious one is the inadequate funding of the health-care system by provincial and federal governments. According to the Fraser Institute, while governments cut funding for health, "they have made it virtually impossible for Canadians to voluntarily pay more for their own health care" and thereby jump to the head of the queue, as those in need of cataract surgery are able to do in Alberta. But it is the complicity of governments in the expansion, not narrowing, of private-sector alternatives, and the increased role of for-profit companies that are creating many of the problems associated with growing queues among lower- and middle-income earners for necessary services. There are no queues for wealthy patients who can afford to go elsewhere for the best care and the shortest waits.

Many businesses supported the use of managed care as a "promising solution" to the problems cited by right-wing commentators from the

Fraser Institute, the C.D. Howe Institute, and other think tanks. The sudden interest of big business in how and which hospitals delivered health care reflected a growing conviction among employers that they were paying more for health and, therefore, should have a larger say in how the system was run. Managed care had helped put U.S. employers in the driver's seat, which was exactly where their Canadian counterparts wanted to be.

Although many employers worried that defining health was "a slippery issue," they demanded more tangible evidence to determine what constituted a medically necessary procedure. Empirical research on what kind of care and which medical procedures were effective and appropriate would "enlarge our knowledge base," employers at a business roundtable sponsored by the Conference Board of Canada said, "and lead to informed decision making on the scope of services to be covered by public health insurance." The federal government, they argued, should create and enforce national standards to measure the efficiency and effectiveness of procedures. Business leaders from some of Canada's largest corporations planned to bring their experience and "keen sense of the process of restructuring" to bear on health-sector renewal, advising hospitals on successful reengineering models and practice guidelines that would support the cost-cutting goals employers wanted to see implemented.[11]

To increase their profile on the subject, powerful voices in the business community began to organize. Citing studies that projected their share of the health bill would increase to over one third by the late 1990s as delisted services made their way onto employee benefits plans, business began to demand a larger influence over how the system operated. Corporate employers never failed to point out that "for decades" they had contributed payroll taxes to support medicare and had provided health and dental benefits plans to millions of workers, giving them additional protection in the event of a major health crisis. Business leaders complained that governments assumed employer-sponsored health plans would pick up coverage for services no longer provided by public insurance. But, they warned bluntly, "it ain't necessarily so, Joe."[12]

Business leaders also grumbled that publicly financed health care had created a perception among Canadians that health services were free, leading workers on supplementary benefits plans to assume extended health coverage was both a right and a necessity. "As people who have some influence on attitudes," the roundtable group told the Conference Board of Canada in 1995, employers should address the "growth of an entitlement mentality" among Canadians who were able to "access the system for any health issue, at any time, in any province" without ever seeing a bill. The management of health care, they insisted, must include a "focus on realigning consumer attitudes" away from such notions of entitlement as well as increased control of "supplier-induced demand." This was a reference to "service suppliers," notably fee-for-service physicians, who "may tend to over-service the customer/patient."[13]

The factors contributing to employers' increased health costs were many. Public plans often were slow, or failed entirely, to respond to the introduction of new medical devices or drugs, causing employees to seek coverage on employer-sponsored plans. Services reduced or cut entirely from public health plans – many because they were not deemed medically necessary – included annual physical and eye exams, ophthalmology services, coverage for foreign students or for family members of temporary foreign workers, out-of-country portability, and dental health programs for children. Many of these were shifted to employer-sponsored benefits plans. Private health plans also felt the impact of new management strategies implemented by hospitals that led to shorter patient turnarounds and early discharges. Such tactics, employers complained (while at the same time supporting them), were increasing employees' use of home care, rehab, and private nursing services and inevitably would raise demands for expanded coverage for these services in supplementary benefit packages. In provinces implementing health-reform initiatives, employers were deep in discussions with provincial and regional authorities about how physiotherapy and other services should be delivered – outside the hospital sector and by private companies such as Columbia Health Care.[14]

But the biggest cost driver was drugs. From 1987 to 1996 the cost of prescription drugs in Canada rose by 93 percent, compared to an increase in the Consumer Price Index of 23.1 percent. Paradoxically, employers complained that the early discharge strategies being implemented by cash-strapped hospitals – strategies they enthusiastically supported – had led to a further shift of costs to business because drugs, covered by public plans as long as patients were hospitalized, were paid for by the employer's plan when the patient was sent home. (The issue of drug costs is covered in detail in chapter 10.)

Along with rising drug costs, the ranks of retired workers on company benefits plans – whose numbers, many employers asserted, were equivalent to or greater than their active workforce – were growing. These factors, plus changing demographics that would see the number of Canadians sixty-five years and older increasing to 20 percent of the population by 2021, all translated "into potentially significant costs to employers in the future." In response, employers began aggressively decreasing benefits to retirees, usually through tough negotiations at the bargaining table with unions.[15]

Employers rise up

Although large employers did not consider the 8.7 percent of payroll spent by U.S. companies on health care to be a "deal-breaker" when considering investments south of the border, they complained bitterly about the 1.4 percent of payroll required to provide extended health coverage to their Canadian employees. Despite their criticism of government cost shifting, employers themselves moved to download health costs to their employees and retired beneficiaries. These tactics were well established in the United States, where the largest employers were able to lock insurers into long-term deals that pegged premium increases as low as 0.01 percent in 1995-96, the lowest rate of increase in thirteen years of tracking by the Department of Labor. One reason for the decline in employers' costs was the shift to managed care plans, which by the mid-1990s counted 73 percent of all covered employees as clients. Another reason companies saved money, and a significant one, was that they were "sharing the costs with the medical users." Large employers – who passed on their costs to workers in the form of higher deductibles and increased monthly co-payments for premiums

– were able to escape the 11 percent increase in benefits plan premiums in 1995 that was charged to smaller businesses with less clout and fewer employees.[16]

The introduction of so-called flexible benefit packages was another cost-saving measure introduced by U.S. employers. Flexible benefits gave employees a "choice" of several plans offering a wider or narrower range of benefits. If employees selected a "deluxe" health plan, the company paid a reduced percentage of the premium, forcing workers to shoulder more of the cost. If a more "cost-effective" but less comprehensive plan was chosen, employee co-payments would be less and companies would save as well, particularly if they exerted pressure on insurers to lower costs in exchange for delivering a large number of clients. "Because we don't have any more money to give them, [employees] have to find ways to do more with less," explained the manager of health-care strategy and programs for the Xerox Corporation. But either way, employees paid the price in higher premiums and deductibles or in increased out-of-pocket expenses for services not covered on their managed care health plans.[17]

The predictable result was an increase of at least $5.5 billion from 1989 to 1996 in employees' health-care costs across the U.S., with further increases projected by the end of the century. A study by Lewin-ICF, a U.S. health consulting firm, for the Service Employees International Union estimated that average family spending on premium co-payments, deductibles, and uninsured medical expenses had risen from $939 in 1980 to $2,303 in 1992, an increase of 145 percent. Employers who argued that health costs threatened their viability and profits entered union negotiations with demands that workers accept higher premium co-payments and deductibles, plus lower wage increases or wage cuts. Health-insurance benefits became "the toughest issue at the bargaining table" by the early 1990s and the number one cause of strikes, despite the fact that benefit payments for employees and their families ceased when the work did.[18]

These patterns were soon spilling over the border. A 1994 study by the Conference Board of Canada found that 80 percent of employers felt they were "paying too much" for health benefits, while many business executives said that rising health costs were threatening to undermine the competitive edge they had enjoyed in the global marketplace before their benefit payments began climbing "at an alarming rate." "How can we justify maintaining jobs in Canada given the very competitive nature of business?" fretted one executive from a U.S. multinational, adding that while benefit costs were significantly lower in Canada than the United States, they were increasing at a faster rate. A survey conducted by Benefits Canada in 1993 to ascertain how employers were responding to rising health and dental costs showed that 30 percent of employers had placed limits on specific items covered under supplementary health plans, while 21 percent did so for dental services, 18 percent increased employees' premium co-payments, 16 percent increased deductibles, and 11 percent reduced the lifetime maximum benefit payouts.[19]

Canadian employers also began promoting flexible benefits plans as an alternative that they said would provide more "choice" to their employees. Unions negotiating collective agreements were now confronted by employer demands for reduced benefits, caps on employer contribution levels, and the use of employer-designated physicians to examine workers claiming sick pay. During the 1980s, workers accepted expanded benefits in lieu of wage increases. But in the 1990s, trade unions were forced to defend those same benefits at the bargaining table while simultaneously campaigning against government cutbacks in health-care funding and delisting. It was not a campaign that employers chose to join. In the fall of 1996, when the United Steelworkers rejected a three-year freeze on health benefits for guards employed by Bradson Security in Ottawa, they were threatened with a lockout, a warning of what was on the horizon for a growing number of Canadian workers.[20]

Educating the workers and organizing the employers

Employers were not only focussed on bargaining tables. Many were convinced that workers abused the system because they were ignorant and unaccountable, while others thought they were simply irresponsible. Large employers viewed workers with condescension and paternalism and believed that most of them simply needed the sensitive guidance of an effective information and communications strategy to understand how important it was to reduce corporate health costs. Partnerships that emphasized education and information, said Alan Cunningham of Suncor Energy, would go a long way towards convincing employees that they had "to accept some accountability." It was not enough that workers paid the lion's share of Canada's $75 billion health bill in the form of taxes, premium co-payments, and out-of-pocket expenditures. Employers wanted them to pay even more, and they were about to get a lot of help from insurers, consultants, private providers, and governments.[21]

The emphasis on education reflected the view that employee resistance to reduced benefits arose because workers were blissfully unaware of the true costs associated with health care and were unable to ascertain their own needs. Employees were not "educated enough to start making [health care] decisions" on their own, said Susan Bird of J. J. McAteer & Associates. Like many other employers, she had personal experience of this. "I see examples every day of plan members who have just followed a long path of completely inappropriate treatment" prescribed by physicians, she said. "So I feel the consumer needs to be taught to take responsibility."

Flexible benefits were one of the most effective ways to educate employees. Said Jean Faber of the Bank of Nova Scotia, "It forces them to learn the value and cost of benefits because up until this point, they've had an entitlement mentality."[22]

But employers encountered a "minefield" of labour relations problems as they introduced "flex plans" and tried to force workers to assume a greater share of health-care costs. Employers were plagued by a range of what they called "attitude problems," including, they said, a stubborn, anachronistic faith among workers that access to health services was a civil right. William Vickers of The Oshawa Group, which employed 18,000 unionized workers, said the differences between a nonunionized and unionized environment could not be underestimated. Unionized employees, he suggested, were stuck in the past and had trouble "getting to newer thinking, more accountable thinking." Workers and their unions still viewed "any reduction [as] a ... takeaway," instead of as a way to increase responsibility and accountability.

As well, many workers were just not ready to make "healthy choices and live a lifestyle that is conducive to long-term well-being." Karen Gordon of National Sea Products in Halifax deplored the fact that "most of the employees who come and complain that a certain asthma medication is not covered is the same employee with a cigarette in their hand." From tobacco giant RJR Macdonald, long known for its concern about public health, Anne Duncan asserted that "we're ... going to flex" because "our costs are just going up and we want employees to become more responsible for their own benefits." John Chiarelli of Coca Cola concurred: "The bottom line today is flex as far as I'm concerned. We, as an employer, cannot afford to go on as we have been," he said. "The bottom line is we're shifting away from corporate responsibility [for health care]." When Canada Trust implemented a "flex plan," said Vic Clive, vice president of human resources, it simply told its 13,000 nonunion employees "that we were about to become facilitators of benefits, not guarantors of benefits." While unionized workers were fighting at the bargaining table to protect their benefits packages, the unorganized had no choice but to accept what employers said was in the best interests of workers.[23]

In 1992, thirteen of Alberta's largest employers formed the Alberta Employer Committee on Health Care (AECHC) at the invitation of William M. Mercer Ltd., a U.S. multinational benefits consulting firm with a Canadian client base of 3000 companies. Several months before issuing its invitation, William M. Mercer had called for "open talks" between governments and business about the "explosive growth in employers' costs for government-managed programs" such as unemployment insurance, pensions, and health care. Dean Connor, head of the company's western region, demanded to know whether "employers [would] have to cut back the benefit programs they sponsor in order to make room in their budgets for the ever-increasing cost of ... social programs" facing government funding cuts. "With increased financial responsibility," he said, "should come a larger role for employers in the design and operation of these programs."[24]

The AECHC – which included household names like Suncor Energy, Nova Corporation, Canada Pipelines, and, needless to say, William M. Mercer – focussed largely on strategies designed to reduce the cost of employer-sponsored benefits plans. But it also broadened its scope to "identify opportunities where employers can help to improve the cost and effectiveness of the health system." To achieve this larger goal it would have to influence the provincial government's health-policy decisions, a task it undertook with vigour. In a brief submitted to Alberta's health minister in December 1993, the group declared its support for cutbacks in the health-care sector but pointed out that employer-sponsored plans were intended merely to supplement, not replace, government programs. The brief recommended that health-care premiums be imposed on seniors who could afford to pay. "It is instructive to note," said the *Financial Post* (which did), "that the recent Alberta budget requires seniors to pay health premiums."[25]

This early success led the employers' group to seek closer ties with the dental and drug industries to more effectively manage skyrocketing costs. According to AECHC member Jack Pilchar, a consultant at William M. Mercer, talks with the Alberta Dental Association proved fruitful. "We told them that if other organizations are restructuring and finding more efficient, better ways of doing business, then perhaps they ought to as well, because employers are not going to continue to sponsor dental plans if costs go up uncontrollably." In 1996, Alberta dentists decided to freeze their fees, the result, said Pilchar, "at least in some small part, of our efforts."

The AECHC was not as successful with the Pharmaceutical Manufacturers Association of Canada (PMAC), which represents U.S.-based drug companies. After "exhaustive discussions" with PMAC about drug-pricing strategies, the AECHC admitted that no action was likely to be forthcoming. Instead, said Pilchar, employers left their meetings with the drug companies armed with useful information about how to restrict employee drug options and negotiate "provider arrangements" with a select group of pharmacies.[26]

Encouraged by these stories, Ontario employers, including Noranda, IBM, Northern Telecom, Dofasco, and Ontario Hydro, decided in 1994 that they would not "sit on the sidelines as crucial decisions about health care are made." Thirty-one of Ontario's largest employers founded the Employer Committee on Health Care-Ontario (ECHO), whose first contribution to the public debate was a demand that pilot studies be initiated on user fees. The group called for hospital closures; wider use of lower-paid health professionals; increased use of information technology to track patients' medical histories, prescription drug use, and diagnostic testing records; and a bonus system for doctors who "discourage over-treatment but encourage preventive care."

While on the surface many of ECHO's proposals sounded rational – after all, who could argue that overtreatment should not be discouraged? – it was the fine print that mattered. Some of ECHO's members had invested heavily in the health industry or sat as directors on the boards of health corporations. Not surprisingly, therefore, they were reluctant to take on the suppliers of health products and services but turned instead to managing the demand side of the equation. Physicians, the group charged, were overtreating or overprescribing because they were "likely to succumb" to pressure from patients. Another problem was employees who would opt for the most expensive drug "touted ... on the Internet as a cure for hangovers and other minor ills," especially "if they can get it for free" in a generous benefits package. "People shop around," said a senior associate at Deloitte and Touche, "but as soon as they're covered by a plan, they don't shop around." Victor Clive, ECHO member and Canada Trust executive, concurred, adding that he would like to see the health-care system function more like the "real marketplace," where consumers had to exercise greater discretion.[27]

ECHO, made up of large employers who provided supplementary benefits to employees, said its members had seen health costs rise by 74 percent between 1990 and 1994 and stated that such increases could not be sustained. Claiming it was "not a slash-and-burn organization," the employers' group said it wanted to "maintain and sustain the comprehensive benefit plans" providing coverage to employees, but "we have to consider costs, or else these will implode." However, while ECHO identified drugs as the biggest expense, the group pointed to new drug therapies, new diseases, increased drug use, and an ageing workforce as the main culprits responsible for rising costs. Like their Alberta counterparts, they spared drug manufacturers any suggestion of culpability. ECHO's strategy was not to take on the drug industry, but rather to transfer the costs to employees through flexible benefits plans – flexible in the sense that workers would be forced "to make choices," "shop smarter," and shoulder a greater share of the cost.[28]

To this end, ECHO said it was using information technology to track employee drug use and was making the data available to "medical researchers" to determine "which medicines deliver the best outcomes" – including the best possible cost-containment outcome. Large employers, in partnership with private insurers, implemented other strategies such as charging employees higher deductibles, discontinuing some benefits, and setting lower payout ceilings on claims. "For employees, the benefit bonanza appears to be over," gushed *Profit* magazine, citing provincial delisting and the "evolutionary component" – ageing baby boomers with more expensive illnesses – as the main reasons for escalating costs.

As the private sector clamoured for a more influential role in healthcare decision making, employers continued to lament their exclusion from the public debate. They found sympathetic ears in many provincial governments and a friendly pipeline in the Canadian media, through which they channelled their solutions to the supposedly health-care-induced debt crisis to an anxious public. One remedy for escalating health costs, embraced by a growing number of Canadian companies that thrust the idea into the centre of their discussions with governments, insurers, and providers, was managed care, "an integrated free-enterprise model for health service delivery developed in the United States."[29]

This idea, as well as the concept of groups like ECHO and AECHC that sponsored private health plans for their workers, was imported directly from the U.S. by Canadian subsidiaries of U.S.-based corporations. For example, the Washington (DC) Business Group on Health (WBGH), founded in 1974 and composed of 194 large employers (most of them Fortune 500 corporations), sponsored private health coverage for over 30 million workers and their families in the United States. Like the many other state-based employer health groups in the U.S., WBGH played an influential role during debates on President Clinton's health-reform initiative. Many of its member companies helped pioneer managed care in order to control benefit costs. In mid-1994, a membership survey conducted by the group reflected a strong desire among large employers "for health reform to be comprehensive and to allow them to remain active purchasers of health care, preserving and building upon the many significant marketplace reforms spearheaded by the private sector." A majority of employers agreed that the "integration of health care providers into organized systems of care" was the most important goal of reform, while 97 percent supported competition "as the best means of controlling overall health spending." Respondents expressed overwhelming support for the application of their solutions to both the public and private sectors. Employers, said WGBH, "recognize that reform of public programs – for which private companies have long borne much of the cost – is necessary to generate the needed revenues for comprehensive coverage."[30]

Large employers also were adamant that the role of government should be to set initial guidelines only. Monitoring the quality of care should be the private sector's responsibility. The federal government, they said, should define the services that health plans must provide and the standards they must meet, including standards for data collection and reporting. Then the private sector must be given responsibility for "establishing and running purchasing pools, collecting and reporting required performance data, and determining cost-sharing" arrangements between employers and employees.

Many of the corporations involved in the Washington group were active in Canada's economy as well, employing hundreds of thousands Canadian workers. William M. Mercer Ltd., Ford, General Motors, IBM, General Electric, the Wyatt Company, the Xerox Corporation, the GTE Corporation, Rockwell International, Dupont, Occidental Petroleum, 3M Corporation, Dow Chemical, Weyerhauser, Honeywell, and Hewlett-Packard were among the managed care champions in North America. Other companies, such as Laidlaw (with 66,000 employees in Canada), were advising their shareholders that they had "initiated a managed health care system in the United States." Laidlaw, a major investor in garbage collection and health care, added, "We expect to cut the rate of increase in overall health care costs by one-third while maintaining high-quality health care for our employees." These employers, both Canada- and U.S.-based, viewed the managed care revolution south of the border in a positive light, unlike tens of millions of

Americans who watched their health benefits deteriorating as HMO profits and executive salaries, stock shares, and bonuses soared.[31]

By 1996, Canadian employers were joining forces with insurance and pharmaceutical firms and consultants to lower the cost of their drug, dental, and disability benefits plans. ECHO member Sandra Dudley, regional marketing manager for Manulife Financial Group benefits, told a Toronto conference on public-private partnerships in January 1997 that ECHO's goal was to "become national" and to enter discussions with governments on delisting services, integrated health-delivery systems, the definition of medically necessary, research, and communications. As major investors in health care, she said, "we are buying a seat at the table," stressing that it was "paramount to have a voice and to influence the direction of health care."[32]

The partnership between employers and the corporate health industry was strengthened by several factors. First and foremost was an ideological conviction that profit making in health care was a legitimate, indeed democratic, right for anyone who was prepared to take a risk (the lower the risk the better) with their investment dollars. All arguments flow from this basic tenet, including the Fraser Institute's strenuous defence of the right of every citizen to voluntarily purchase the health care that they need – or don't need.

Another important factor was the increased investment capital flowing from the corporate community to the health industry, not to provide quality health care, but rather because the return on investment was promising, at least for the foreseeable future. Many governments were no longer committed to maintaining current levels of spending on health care, and investors from diverse sectors of the economy – from mining to manufacturing – were flocking to Bay or Wall Street for shares in promising health companies.

And finally, the corporate sector is composed of relatively few people. They sit on corporate boards together, codirecting the activities of their investee companies. They organize alliances and associations to campaign, organize, and lobby in support of their shared interests. In addition, interlocking directorships among executives and investors from companies active across the economy are surprisingly common in Canada. Alcan, Corel Corporation, Miramar Mining, the Royal Bank, the Sherritt Group, IBM, the Toronto *Star*, Laidlaw, the Sun Corporation (owner of the *Financial Post*), Ontario Hydro, and many other familiar names are involved in Canada's health-care industry either through direct investments or through interlocking directorships. Many of these companies are also active in the economies of other countries, most notably the United States, where the introduction of managed care and other private-sector solutions saved them money.

The problems created in the health-care system by government underfunding and cutbacks are hurting Canadian patients and their families. Health care is costing individuals more as they are forced to seek remedies from the private, for-profit companies stepping into the breach. The impact in some parts of Canada is reflected in health statistics. The steep cuts in Alberta's publicly funded health system has resulted in the closure of both urban and rural hospitals, the expansion of corporations such as Columbia Health Care, and the establishment of Canada's first for-profit hospital. The province led the move towards increased private-sector alternatives during the 1990s and now Albertans, especially those in rural areas, are seeing infant mortality rates as high as 10.6 deaths per 1000 live births, compared to a national average of 6.3 deaths per 1000 live births.[33]

NINE

Managing
Care

By the end of 1997, employer health-care committees were up and running in Alberta, Ontario, British Columbia, and Québec, all with similar goals and objectives. At the top of the agenda was the development
of a long-term plan to decrease the amount of money employers were
spending on health care, both in the form of corporate taxes to support
publicly funded health care and premiums paid to insurers for supplementary benefits. Key to this objective was a strategy to wean Canadians from what employers called "the entitlement mentality," which
they said was particularly rampant among working people who had
been "trained and educated ... to expect quality with high cost." In
addition, employers wanted to decrease premiums for workers' compensation by reducing the cost of medical services for injured workers
and the time these workers spent recuperating.[1]

Big business had concluded that one path to saving money – and to
securing increased productivity and higher profits – was managed
care. Another path was tighter management by employers of the 1.4
percent of payroll allocated to health and dental benefits. This would
involve a "vigorous nation-wide push to shift the responsibility of

health care to the party that can have the most impact on outcomes" – the individual. Health care, said employers during roundtable discussions sponsored by Benefits Canada, could be managed if the right ingredients were assembled. The elements in an employer-managed health-care program included flexible benefits plans; higher "participation rates" by employees in the form of increased co-payments and deductibles; the use of information technology to track how, and how much, employees used health services; and tighter control of pharmacy, dental, disability and workers' compensation benefits.

If the strategy for introducing flexible benefits plans was causing problems, especially at bargaining tables, employers were making more headway with company-sponsored employee counselling programs, long-term disability (LTD) claims, and workers' compensation. In these endeavours, information technology was proving to be an indispensable management tool, employers said, enabling them to use data on employee sick time and disability claims "to manage the future." In all provinces, employers were groaning about "out of control" costs associated with increased absenteeism and workers' compensation claims. Many economists credited workforce downsizing and more overtime with the increase in accidents, workload, stress, and family breakdown. But many employers chose to invest in absence and disability management programs rather than decreasing the high workload levels brought on by workforce reductions.[2]

Many tactics focussed on the minutiae of individual employee habits and elaborate methods to control them. One employer surveyed by Ernst & Young in 1996, for example, collected data on each employee's absence due to illness, recording its cause, length, dates, etc., and placed the information in a computerized "employee profile." The employer had invested heavily in the system so it could track "any correlation of casual absences with days before and after statutory holidays," using the information "to substantially improve the absence management program." Employers stepped up what they referred to as "early intervention," in which "there is constant contact with the employee during the period of disability" or absence. While many workers charged this was a form of harassment, employers were determined to pursue their strategies, "whether the cause of disability is occupational or non-occupational."[3]

Tensions between unions and employers were increasing because the employers' strategy often was to control employees' behaviour rather than to improve the health and safety of the work environment. Unions criticized employers who preferred to "manage disability" rather than invest in injury prevention, while employers argued against premium increases to meet compensation and health-care expenses resulting from accidents, occupational diseases, and disabilities incurred in unsafe workplaces. In 1993 the nation's annual bill for workers injured on the job reached $7.5 billion, most of it paid by employers. Ignoring their own rhetoric about increasing employee accountability and responsibility for health care, however, many employers denied their own accountability for workplace accidents and injuries and failed to take responsibility for prevention. Privately managed care promised a less costly alternative, and workers' compensation offered a window of opportunity.

Workers' comp in Canada

Canada's workers' compensation system is funded by employers who pay an assessment or premium based on the injury record of the industry in which they do business, the injury record of the individual company, and the company's number of employees. Workers' compensation is known as a shared risk, or collective liability, fund. Put more simply, employers pool their resources to fund wage replacement, retraining, and medical services for workers injured on the job, while workers forego the right to sue employers for injuries incurred in the workplace, even if the employer is at fault. Employers and employees have an equal number of representatives on provincial Workers' Compensation Boards (WCBs) that collect employer premiums and administer the fund, and that function as agencies of the government. Similar businesses are placed into the same rate groups and their premiums are determined by an industry safety classification system that is periodically adjusted. When a worker is injured, the WCB pays his or her wages until the individual returns to work. Rehabilitation and other required services are provided by both the public and private health-care systems and paid for by the WCB, while vocational training or retraining may be funded and provided directly by the Board. Thus, while Boards are privately funded by employers, they are publicly accountable institutions with premium assessment and wage replacement levels established and regulated by the province. The main costs incurred by the compensation system are for wage replacement, medical services, and retraining.

Both workers and employers have benefitted from the workers' compensation system, which came into existence in most provinces around the time of World War I. Since the late 1980s, however, as government cutbacks reduced hospital and other medical services and increased waiting lists, there were an increasing number of complaints from employers across the country who said that the reductions were hampering efforts to get injured or disabled employees off wage replacement and back into the workforce on a timely basis. These concerns were shared by injured workers, who faced enormous challenges when they confronted the workers' compensation system, beginning with delays in getting the care they needed.

This was often where the common ground between workers and employers ended. Getting workers off wage replacement was the overriding concern of employers – it was, in fact, more important than any other aspect of workplace injury, including the injured worker's readiness to return to work. For workers, lengthy delays in assessments, treatment, and retraining could threaten their chances of a full recovery and of ever returning to a normal work life.

Injured workers receive two types of benefits from the workers' compensation system. The first is in the form of cash payments, a percentage of net or gross income established by the province. The second benefit is in the form of medical care and hospitalization. Workers who are unable to return to the jobs in which their injury occurred also are entitled to vocational retraining. Compensation rates in many Canadian provinces are significantly more generous than those in the privately run and unregulated workers' compensation system in the United States. In 1990, benefit levels in Ontario, for example, were four-and-a-half times higher than the U.S. national average, while in British Columbia they were five times higher. In addition, more workers in Canada are entitled to compensation coverage than their U.S. counterparts. Studies have found that unionized workers are more likely than unorganized workers to receive compensation benefits, in part because unions act on behalf of their members within the workers' comp system to ensure benefits are extended. Such differences might suggest the cost of compensation is greater in Canada than in the United States, but the opposite is true. In a 1998 study, compensation experts Terry Thomason and John Burton found that compensation costs were between 47 percent and 64 percent lower in B.C. than in the U.S., while Ontario's costs were from 26 percent to 43 percent less. One reason for the gap, said the study's authors, could be traced to Canada's "provincial monopoly" of state-run workers' compensation systems, a system that operates in only six U.S. states. Another reason, and an important one, was Canada's publicly run, largely nonprofit, health-care system. In Canada's workers' compensation system, health-care costs accounted for 26 percent of the total benefit package compared to almost 41 percent in the United States. Despite such dramatic evidence, employers continued to insist that the provision of medical services by for-profit companies, as well as a market-driven system of workers' compensation, was more efficient and less costly.[4]

Employers were prime targets of both the private insurance industry and corporate health companies and were as vulnerable to promises of cost savings as the average citizen. In addition, many employers and workers expressed legitimate frustrations about lengthy waiting times for injured workers. This led to employer demands for "queue jumping" so that injured workers could access surgery, rehabilitation, or other needed services and return to work more quickly. But many provincial governments, backed by the public, were reluctant to institute a "two-tiered" plan, with one tier catering to patients covered by public health insurance and another serving injured workers covered by workers' compensation. As governments continued to cut back funding for hospitals, and as hospitals, in turn, closed beds and outpatient rehab services, the workers' compensation system and employers turned increasingly to the corporate sector for solutions.

This pattern escalated in the early 1990s, when more and more employers began seeking out private providers who were prepared to meet the employers' demand that injured employees return to work quickly. In response, medical assessment companies began springing up, particularly in Ontario, offering "rapid medical attention" services to employers. These companies contracted with an employer to steer an injured worker through the medical marketplace and back to work as soon as possible. The companies recruited doctors who wanted to increase their revenues outside the public insurance system through private billings, and organized them into "specialist-referral" or "preferred provider" networks. The assessment service would refer employees to a doctor in the network; if this particular doctor was not available, another one was sure to be. Since network specialists could earn up to twice as much treating patients referred by the assessment company as they could treating a patient with the same problem covered by the public health plan, most doctors made sure they were available. An injured worker would be treated and returned to work more quickly, the employer would reduce the amount paid for wage replacement, and the assessment company and network physician would pocket a tidy sum of money. Unfortunately, patients who were not injured on the job and who were not referred by the assessment company would be bumped to the end of the line.[5]

Such practices were completely legal. Medical assessment companies, employers, and enterprising doctors had discovered the fine print in the Canada Health Act: the "Exclusion Paragraph." The Exclusion Paragraph exempts the treatment of job-related injuries and illnesses from the criteria of the Act if the patient is covered by employer-paid workers' compensation benefits. Simply, public health plans do not provide 24-hour coverage for workers if they are covered by a workers' compensation insurance plan when they are in the workplace. An increasing number of employers, physicians, and private companies were diving through this loophole as quickly as possible.

While many advocates of market medicine credit the queue jumping enabled by the Exclusion Paragraph with "freeing up" the public system, others disagree. "If you're standing in line at a movie theatre and someone in a white fox coat hurries to the head of the line and goes inside and calls back over their shoulder, 'See, the line is shorter now,' would you believe it?" asked Dr. Philip Berger, a family physician and critic of the medical establishment.[6]

Exempt from the criteria of the Canada Health Act, provinces can require that workers' compensation insurance be administered on a nonprofit basis or can allocate the responsibility to private, for-profit insurers that operate under provincial regulations. Since workers' compensation insurance is not governed by the principles of the Act, it operates parallel to public health plans. Like medicare, it has achieved cost efficiencies with services available from publicly funded, nonprofit providers. But the closure of hospital outpatient rehab services and the expansion of rehab services in the for-profit sector are placing upward pressure on costs borne not only by public health plans, but by the workers' compensation system as well, particularly as the incidence of workplace accidents and injuries has continued to climb.

However, employers charged that overly generous benefit levels, rather than increased use of for-profit medical services, were the reason Canada's workers' compensation system was "swamped by debt" and threatened by "unfunded liabilities," a term used liberally in the war of words. Unfunded liability was a phrase employed to conjure up images of a debt-ridden, poorly managed, soon-to-be bankrupt workers' compensation system. But the term referred to the fact there was an inadequate amount of money in the current account to pay for costs projected to be incurred in the future. If a parent, for example, had an "unfunded educational liability," she would lack enough money in her account today to pay the costs of educating her child in ten or twenty years' time. This calculation assumed that the parent – or the workers' compensation system – would cease contributing money to the fund in the intervening years. Despite such thin arguments, fears of a pending disaster in workers' compensation escalated among employers and workers alike.

The employers' bitter and often acrimonious complaints about costs persuaded some provinces that cutbacks were easier to manage than increased premiums for workers' compensation. Reports and studies produced by the Insurance Bureau of Canada, consultants, and private insurers all pointed to skyrocketing assessments, "strange-but-true" anecdotes of system abuses, excessive benefits, and ineffective health programs as the reasons for cost increases. Bending to pressure from powerful employer groups, some provinces began legislating reduced benefit levels and other entitlements in order to force employees to return to work more quickly. These actions served to offload the medical costs of workplace injury to other health plans – both public and private – since these would continue to support ongoing treatment of workers. It also shifted costs from the business community to injured workers, many of whom carried the burden of continued rehabilitation or displacement. At the same time, most provinces failed to introduce legislation to ensure employers invested more heavily in accident prevention.

It was consultants that provided worried employers with the most satisfactory solutions. Multinational consulting firms such as Ernst & Young designed total disability management programs to meet employers' needs, uniting "all facets of a company's health benefits, including wellness, workers' comp, short- and long-term disability, medical benefits and health and family services" into one "seamless delivery system." In this scenario, workers would be covered by an employer-sponsored, twenty-four-hour benefits plan that would oversee the provision of all the health care employers felt would be needed by workers and their families, whether they were injured on the job or contracted an illness at school or the shopping mall. This was care managed by employers and private insurers instead of by individuals in consultation with the general practitioners of their choosing. Described as "integrated health services," these strategies promised to help employers consolidate their control over how, and how much, those services were used, who provided them, and at what cost.[7]

Controlling the injured and disabled, who employers said tended to overuse medical services and who, left to themselves, would no doubt view their time of recuperation as a paid holiday, required an effort called "demand management." According to one consultant, this was not a prevention or wellness strategy. The "overall intent is to reduce utilization, not illness," by looking at the whole picture, including lost productivity due to injury. Demand management depended on information systems that provided data on each employee's use of health-care services and enabled the employer and the insurer to oversee "workers' comp professionals [who may] fool themselves into thinking costs have been reduced just by transferring costs" to another part of the health-care system, particularly long-term disability. Checks and balances on the demand for health services, integrated into a total dis-ability management program, said another consultant, allowed compa-nies "to reduce the costs stemming from unnecessary utilization and get people back on the job sooner."[8]

Managing care in this way was the key, not to improving health and safety in the workplace, but to minimizing the costs associated with not doing so. It was the right solution for employers, consultants, and insurers, one they hoped would bring higher productivity and higher profits. But it was absolutely the wrong answer for people facing risk at work who were one paycheque away from losing the family home – or were struggling to achieve a dignified route back to wellness and back to work.

Liberty and managed rehabilitation

Workers' compensation is the Achilles heel of Canada's health-care system. Exempt from the criteria of the Canada Health Act, provinces are free to assign the provision of insured services to workers' com-pensation boards or to private insurers. Compensation boards, in turn, are free to seek the full spectrum of hospital and rehabilitation services from either publicly funded, nonprofit providers or from private, for-profit companies. The closure or reduction of hospital outpatient ser-vices in the early 1990s has led to unacceptably long waiting times in most provinces for rehabilitation services. The adage "time is money" is the main principle guiding compensation boards, whose chief inter-est is getting workers off wage replacement and who are turning to private rehab companies that promise to get the injured back on the job in record time.

These factors have contributed to a near-complete transformation of outpatient rehabilitation during the last ten years. What once was a nonprofit service delivered by hospitals is now largely a profit-generating business dominated increasingly by a handful of companies like Columbia Health Care. In Alberta and Ontario the rehab industry is moving beyond the delivery of outpatient services. In alliance with other like-minded partners – and in direct competition with nonprofit hospitals – rehab companies are staking out territory in the workers' comp market, a market that includes the provision of inpatient surgical and acute-care services. In addition, vertical integration of the rehab industry in the form of mergers and acquisitions is eliminating small, independent providers and expanding the reach of many U.S.-based companies into Canada's health sector. This is leading to a rapid cross-border amalgamation of the industry and the creation of an integrated North American market.

But integration is not only taking place within the industry and over the border. The insurance industry is targeting both the workers' comp business and rehab services in a strategy known as horizontal integration. This kind of integration takes place when companies merge across traditional corporate boundaries – in this case, when insurance companies merge with rehab providers. With support from many large employers, insurers have mounted an aggressive assault on the workers' compensation system in Canada and are promoting an integrated, managed care approach to the delivery of rehab services on both sides of the border. The strategies being implemented in the United States by workers' compensation insurers, therefore, are of particular relevance to Canadians.

One insurer in particular is moving swiftly to secure a foothold in the workers' comp and rehab markets. Liberty Health (see chapter 5) waded into the troubled waters of Canada's workers' compensation system in the mid-1990s. Its parent, Boston-based Liberty Mutual Group, was the leading workers' compensation insurer in the United States. The options and choices outlined in a series of widely distributed reports sponsored by the company drew generously from its experience in the United States, where workers' compensation is state regulated but privately insured, as are complementary rehabilitation services. Like the Canadian system, workers' comp in the U.S. originally was based on a tradeoff in which workers forfeited the right to sue employers for injuries incurred in the workplace. While this principle has been eroded, U.S. employers are the sole payers of private insurance premiums that provide their injured employees with income replacement, medical and rehabilitation services, and vocational training for alternative employment.

In the U.S., workers' compensation is a growing and highly profitable business for private insurers, who manage the care provided to injured workers on behalf of employers seeking cost reductions through lower and fewer benefits, early return-to-work programs, shared employer-employee contributions, injury prevention, and claims administration. But according to a report in *Canadian Business* magazine, private insurance has produced "dismal results" in the U.S., where employers in most states pay "at least as much as Canadian firms for half the benefits to workers – and face litigation, to boot." Between 1985 and 1993, U.S. workers' compensation costs rose more than 75 percent a year, spurring a state-by-state employers' campaign for legislative reforms aimed at reducing benefit payments, tightening eligibility requirements, and lowering medical costs. These efforts were supported by the workers' comp insurers, who had experienced several years of low profit margins because even premium increases that averaged two to three times the rate of inflation could not keep pace with skyrocketing medical costs. The resulting reforms, combined with the general slow-down of medical care inflation in the mid-1990s, stemmed the increases in state-set workers' comp premiums for larger employers. But many compensation experts noted with dismay that "in an era marked by improved corporate performance, productivity growth, quality improvements, and high profits, workplace safety has deteriorated." They warned that employers who continued to turn their backs on improving workplace safety would see a return of spiralling compensation costs.[9]

Liberty's key sales pitch to Canada's business sector was "managed care on an integrated basis," an approach it said would save employers money and, needless to say, provide the insurer with a new and lucrative source of revenue. It was not unreasonable to ask how two apparently contradictory aims could be achieved simultaneously. What was it specifically about Liberty's managed care scheme that promised cost reductions to employers and profits to the insurer, particularly when the cost drivers – expensive technology, an ageing population, occupational injuries and disease, and public to private sector downloading – were not predicted to ease up?

The answer to this question was to be found in the United States. Described as one of the "most aggressive players" in the U.S. compensation marketplace, Liberty Mutual spent the early 1990s diversifying its operations. These efforts led the corporation into the "provider market" in the U.S. in a bid to create an integrated health-delivery system in which it would control all aspects of workers' compensation, "from writing insurance policies to providing actual care." In 1994 Liberty began implementing a long-term plan to increase its hold on the workers' comp market with the purchase of twelve occupational rehabilitation centres across the United States to treat its workers' compensation and disability insurance claimants.

Liberty's plan called for the construction of huge rehabilitation centres in different locations throughout the U.S. These would offer a range of rehab and assessment services, including substance abuse monitoring, and staff would "gather data on the management of ... claims to determine optimum treatment and case management strategies."[10] Liberty's strategy differed from that of other insurers, who formed alliances with networks of managed care providers, negotiated costs, and influenced treatment protocols. Instead, Liberty was planning to become both insurer and provider with controlling interest in a nationwide chain of rehab providers. This would position the insurer in the "occupational injury niche of the market," offering cost reductions of between 10 percent and 20 percent to employers who sent their injured workers to facilities designated by Liberty. "If you cannot do something like that in the latter part of the 1990s," said Liberty Mutual vice-president Thomas Ramey, "you can't be in business."[11]

Liberty moved quickly to implement its strategy. In January 1995 it formed the Atlantic Health Group to handle ownership of its new rehabilitation facilities. By mid-1996, after a flurry of acquisitions in the eastern U.S., the Atlantic Health Group was the leading provider of occupational health and rehabilitation services in the eastern United States. The group offered workers' compensation injury and illness treatment; physiotherapy and rehab services; occupational, sports, and environmental health services; and medical assessments. The company's "comprehensive workers compensation managed care product" was tailored to meet the needs of employers. "The most significant result of a workplace injury," said Liberty, "is the potential loss of a valuable asset" for employers who suffered from lost productivity, incurred costs for training and paying replacement workers, and shouldered the cost of workers' compensation payments.[12]

Liberty's plan to reduce employer costs and secure high profits entailed far more than just holding the line on the costs of medical care. "This is not about controlling any one area of business," Ramey said. "The idea is to control the entire continuum of the workers' compensation process." Control over how injured workers were assessed, who treated them, and for how long was the key to what Liberty referred to as its "early return to work strategy." Put more bluntly, the sooner workers were off wage replacement, the more money the insurer would make. It was a strategy that was working: net premium income for the company increased from $5.3 billion in 1994 to about $6 billion a year later, while its underwriting losses in workers' compensation were slashed, due in large measure to "effective loss prevention and managed care techniques." Liberty also recorded a remarkable increase in the value of its assets, which rose from $20.6 billion to over $65 billion by 1996, stark testimony to its success on the acquisition trail.[13]

Liberty Mutual wanted to apply these successful strategies in the global market. The company's diversification scheme included the founding of Liberty International to provide insurance and occupational health and safety services in other countries, notably in Canada, Mexico, Japan, Latin America, and Europe. Although Liberty was established in Canada during the 1930s, it began aggressively branching out into the Canadian health-care market in 1993, with the acquisition of the Premier Treatment and Health Management Centre, a company rechristened International Managed Health Care by its new 70 percent majority shareholder. Based in Toronto, IMHC began to expand to treat auto accident victims who required outpatient rehabilitation services in Mississauga, Toronto, Hamilton, and Scarborough.

The cuts in health funding in Ontario helped Liberty by forcing patients to seek alternatives to outpatient rehabilitation services that were disappearing as the hospital sector downsized. Equally important, the introduction of no-fault insurance in 1990, described as a "boon to [private] clinics because it provided large payments for treatments," placed new restrictions on patients' right to sue. When private insurers offered guarantees that people injured in auto accidents would receive coverage for rehabilitation, the private rehab market began to sprout. Liberty was the first insurer to "jump directly into the fray," using IMHC to "spearhead the introduction of many programs already offered in the U.S., where the concept of managed care has been growing for years."[14]

But Liberty's U.S. acquisition strategy was proving to be more difficult in the Canadian market. In March 1996 Liberty launched an apparently rancorous bid to purchase the remaining 30 percent of minority shares held by IMHC's founders, Rich Ferreira and Rocco Lofranco. When negotiations reached an impasse, Liberty abruptly announced that it could no longer support the company under its current structure and, more to the point, it was not "prepared to finance 100 percent of the company's bills, while only owning 70 percent of the shares." The move sent IMHC into receivership after the company's bank demanded repayment of a $12 million debt in May. By late summer, Columbia Health Care Inc., Canada's largest private rehab company (see chapter 6), bought IMHC, boosting the number of clinics in its chain of for-profit rehab centres to thirty-two.[15]

This failed effort in the rehab market was a temporary setback for Liberty. The company's beeline into the potentially lucrative workers' comp business in Canada was buttressed by its 1995 purchase of Ontario Blue Cross. From this vantage point it was able to play an active role in the emerging debates about how injured and disabled workers should be treated. In June 1995 Liberty International released a study that proposed a substantial redesign of the workers' compensation system and outlined its unique ability to deliver the services employers required. "In commissioning this study," said Liberty International's Canadian president, Brian Johnston, "I saw it as a means of contributing to public consideration of the choices that we, as a country, must make in shaping the future of workers' compensation in Canada."

When Liberty released its five-volume report entitled "Unfolding Change," Ontario and Alberta were listening with interest to industry proposals for a streamlined, efficient, and cheaper method of insuring against workplace accidents. In an introductory comment to the study's outline, Johnston candidly admitted that his company had "a long-term business interest as to the direction workers' compensation reform ultimately takes. I believe that a viable, workable and responsive system requires private sector participation and, based on Liberty's vast experience in workers' compensation in the United States ... , we probably have a place on that spectrum in Canada when the time comes."[16]

Liberty's workers' compensation system of the future would be market-based and competitive, providing integrated medical, related health and return-to-work services. The company claimed that its reforms were "founded on injury prevention as a first priority." However, the few proposals on this subject centred on suggestions that employers with good safety records "must be given more immediate and meaningful rewards" and provided with "greater incentives ... for safety and injury prevention."

If employers needed rewards to motivate them to establish safe and healthy workplaces, injured workers needed the threat of lower benefit levels to get them back on the job as quickly as possible. The benefits provided to injured workers, Liberty concluded, were too generous and tended to discourage them from returning to work as soon as possible. It was a perspective that portrayed injured workers as people who wanted to milk the system for as long and as much as possible – a situation that could be addressed with the threat of reduced income and drastic cutbacks in workers' comp benefits across Canada. This was just the after-the-injury cost-reduction strategy that employers wanted to hear.

In Liberty's plan, rehab companies, insurers, and employers would achieve what it called an "alignment of incentives." The incentive was the promise of increased revenues and healthy profits for employers, insurers, and the rehab industry. All of this could be achieved with "the introduction of competitive pricing for workers' compensation services." Competitive pricing would keep everyone on their toes:

rehab providers would be motivated to maintain high-quality services, insurers would want to hold premiums in check, and employers
would shop around for the lowest cost alternatives to designing safer
work environments. Unfortunately, such an alignment of incentives
would also provide insurers and rehab companies with an interest in
maintaining, rather than reducing, the high rate of accidents and
injuries in the workplace, since neither would see a healthy return on
investment if the number of occupational injuries decreased.

Liberty followed its cross-Canada report on workers' compensation
with a paper presented to the government of Ontario, which was
reviewing options for reform of its workers' compensation system
early in 1996. The paper was critical of the Ontario Workers' Compensation Board (OWCB), which "on a comparative basis ... does not fare
well in many of the categories measured." In particular, Liberty
pointed to the OWCB's $11.5 billion unfunded liability, the severity
and duration of claims by injured workers, the high level of benefits
paid, poor claims management, and poor standards of service. Describing the OWCB pejoratively as a "monopoly organization" subject to
"inherent bureaucratic inertia," Liberty outlined its proposals for a
"mixed enterprise model of competition" embracing "integrated,
managed health and return-to-work care for injured workers" and the
"effective implementation of 'best practices' or protocols."[17]

Calling for increased efficiencies and effectiveness, the company
launched a small-is-beautiful attack on the "current public monopoly
system." The OWCB suffered from a "limited responsiveness" to
injuries, Liberty charged, because it was hampered by a large bureau-
cracy employing 4600 people to serve most of the 3.3 million employees covered by workers' compensation insurance. Never mind that the
OWCB's large proportions paled in comparison to Liberty's own mammoth size, its vast global reach, and its 23,000 employees in 450 offices
worldwide. Nor would Liberty have cared to point out that it was one
of fifty-three private carriers in Ontario employing 3500 people to
serve a smaller – in fact, much smaller – percentage of covered employees than the "public monopoly."[18]

Notwithstanding this contradiction, Liberty proposed that the
OWCB be broken up into a "number of functional responsibilities."

Instead of being handled by a single entity like OWCB, which was made up of employer and employee representatives, these responsibilities could be taken up by private, for-profit entities. In this new structure – described as a "recasting of roles across the spectrum of workers' compensation, administration and service" – the OWCB would be reduced to "competing with private carriers for the province's workers' compensation business."[19]

The managed care emphasis inherent in the company's scheme would allow Liberty to begin building a foundation that mirrored its U.S. workers' comp operations. Placing control of all medical, related health, and return-to-work services in the hands of a privately run workers' compensation insurer would minimize the insurer's costs by imposing on workers specified treatment protocols designed to move them as quickly as possible back to work, thus lowering wage replacement payments. But protocols that aimed to remove workers from the compensation rolls often ignored the goal of returning workers expeditiously to good health.

Liberty's proposals struck a cord with employers, but they worried union activists involved in occupational health and safety. The company acknowledged the fact that managed care involved "protocols inconsistent with the principle of unlimited physician choice by the employee," a matter that "must be clearly dealt with at the outset." If injuries could be shown to have originated outside the workplace, workers would not be entitled to wage replacement and the cost of medical services would fall on the public health plan rather than the compensation insurer. Most doctors, Liberty said, did not use appropriate treatment protocols, had "little knowledge of the workplace ... and [were] not in a position to assess if injuries [were] work-related." Liberty's solution to these problems was the "empowered case manager" who would act as a "quarterback," overseeing physicians and other providers to get the injured and disabled off what was viewed by many employers as a benefits gravy train.[20]

If this view of working people was unforgiving, Liberty's plan for small employers was only slightly more generous. Premium rates in a competitive system, the company admitted, could lead "to the possibility that a significant group of employers will face substantially higher rates." This group of mainly small businesses would compose a "residual market" – employers who would be unwilling or unable to pay higher premiums and who private carriers would not voluntarily insure because of the potentially higher risks involved. These smaller and high-risk businesses could always fall back on the OWCB as the insurer-of-last-resort.

When the Ontario government unveiled its long-awaited plan for OWCB reform in mid-1995, the response from the insurance industry was mixed. The package, described by Mike Harris's Conservative government as a "difficult but necessary measure," would reduce benefit levels for injured workers from 90 percent to 85 percent of take-home pay. Eligibility rules would be tightened, compensation for chronic stress would be eliminated entirely, and workers suffering from chronic pain would see their benefits reduced. But the reform package was not all bad news: the government reduced employers' assessment rates to the OWCB by 5 percent, despite their concerns about the unfunded liability.

The Insurance Bureau of Canada (IBC), representing insurers across the country, had lobbied for a complete privatization of the OWCB during 1995. While it held little hope of achieving that goal immediately, it was confident that eventually workers' comp would simply be another line of insurance available from the private sector. The IBC responded favourably, therefore, to the Conservative government's reform package, which the IBC's Ontario representative, Stan Griffin, said took the province a "closer step" towards OWCB privatization.[21]

Liberty International was not as enthusiastic about the government's reform package as others in the industry were. Bill Wilkerson of Liberty criticized the Conservatives' plan because it failed to address disability management and the critical goal of getting workers off wage replacement with early-return-to-work strategies. The government, he said, was not ready to introduce competition to the injured workers business. But he looked on the bright side and added that there likely was room for the private sector to pick up outsourced claims and case management, something other insurers were not well equipped to handle. "We need an approach to claims management that works closely with the case manager," he said. "The traditional [insurance] approach may not be right. We need to bring down the costs ... by a process that gets the person back to work."[22]

Liberty's energetic Canadian campaign reflected the company's global approach and Canada's place in the corporate plan. The company's position on a privatized and integrated Canadian workers' compensation industry was in keeping with Liberty's diversification efforts in the United States and its strategy to export its services to other countries – though Canada was not just any other country. In fact, it was not really another country at all, as Liberty viewed its Canadian business as a part of its U.S. operation. The company had no intention of adjusting its U.S. style to fit what it saw as an outdated and restrictive nonprofit Canadian health-care system. Instead, the system would have to adjust to Liberty and its plans to bring an integrated American model for workers compensation and rehabilitation to eager Canadian employers.

Exclusion and the for-profit tier

The workers' compensation system was opening doors to the insurance industry, and for-profit rehabilitation companies and hospitals were not prepared to sit idly by and watch. They wanted a piece of the action, too. Advocates of a parallel, for-profit tier in the health-care system were relieved to see that such a goal might be within reach without their having to take on the sacred principles of the Canada Health Act.

The first real test of the Act's exclusion paragraph for workers' compensation came in September 1997, with the opening of a $6 million, 37-bed, for-profit hospital in Calgary. The Health Resources Group, put together by a group of investors, former regional health officials, and physicians, took over the third floor of the former Grace Hospital, which had recently been closed by the province. The company's decision to open in Calgary was based on a number of factors, including the closure of three acute-care hospitals, the elimination of more than 1500 hospital jobs from 1993 to 1997, and spending cuts of $143 million to the city's health-care budget during the same period. In addition, Albertans had seen a 20 percent reduction in the province's health-care budget, leading regional health officials to look at the potential for public-private partnerships with for-profit providers.

Founded in Alberta in 1995, within two years HRG had developed an ambitious business plan and strong ties with the province's ruling Conservative Party. It also had a network of business allies in the health industry, as well as among Alberta's employers. HRG was training its eye on the workers' compensation market and on employers who wanted top-of-the-line services delivered outside the increasingly clogged hospital system where, they complained, injured workers were placed on lengthy waiting lists. The company's plan included the establishment of a for-profit chain of hospitals, beginning in Calgary and expanding rapidly to locations in Edmonton, Toronto, and Vancouver. HRG planned to offer, among other things, orthopedic, general, and plastic surgery; inpatient and outpatient medical and rehabilitation services; and services to support clinical drug trials. "Wherever possible," its 1997 business plan said, "these services will be offered in a non-union environment."[23]

HRG brought together some powerful backers, including executives from two health multinationals: Sun Healthcare (parent of Columbia Health Care) and MDS. Columbia had received nearly $7.5 million in business from the Alberta Workers' Compensation Board in 1996, and was on good terms with the board's chief executive offficer, John Cowell. In December 1997, after five years at the helm of the WCB, Cowell resigned with a retirement package worth almost $600,000, in addition to his annual salary of $366,000. Less than four months later, he was working as a consultant for Columbia, a key player in Alberta's new private hospital.[24]

Frank King, who chaired the 1988 Calgary Winter Olympics, was a major investor in the for-profit hospital and was named its chief executive officer. The head of a venture capital firm called Metropolitan Investment, King had strong links to the petroleum industry and was the president and CEO of the Inmark Group, Avanti Petroleums Ltd., and Cambridge Environmental Systems, Inc. He also sat as a director on a number of corporate boards, including the Sherritt Group and the parent company of Canada's premiere business newspaper, the *Financial Post*. The head of HRG's board was Peter Burgener, an architect, former chair of the Calgary District Hospital Group, and husband of a member of Ralph Klein's government.[25]

The president of HRG was Jim Saunders, former chief operating officer with the Calgary Regional Health Authority, the body that oversaw the city's hospital services. During his term at CRHA, Saunders supported the participation of for-profit companies in the delivery of a range of health and diagnostic services including nursing and home care, cataract surgery, rehabilitation, and palliative care. When the private hospital was announced, Saunders promised it would offer a broad range of acute-care services and would have three operating rooms available for inpatient and day surgery. HRG was confident that it would be awarded contracts by the CRHA and other regional health bodies to provide patients with more "choice" in hospital services. But HRG expected its first big contract would be with the Alberta Workers Compensation Board, with an annual budget of $73.5 million to spend in the health-care system. Saunders reassured Albertans that HRG intended "to fully conform with every aspect of the Canada Health Act," meaning that the company could dip liberally into the WCB's fund and remain on the right side of the law.[26]

In addition to Saunders and Burgener, the company's directors included Dr. Stephen Miller, a cofounder of HRG and its chief medical officer. Miller was also the chief of orthopedic surgery at the Foothills Hospital and an associate clinical professor at the University of Calgary. Tom Saunders (no relation to Jim), vice-chair and director of HRG, cofounded a private rehabilitation centre with Miller that was taken over by U.S.-based Sun Healthcare Group, which then appointed him to head up the multinational's Canadian division. Dr. William Cochrane, another director, was a former dean of medicine, former president of the University of Calgary, and former deputy minister of health services for Alberta. More importantly, Cochrane headed up a health venture capital fund owned by multinational health conglomerate MDS Inc. MDS managed the Canadian Medical Discoveries Fund, another venture capital project based in Ottawa, which had contributed $2 million in start-up capital to the for-profit hospital.

HRG insisted that one of its main contributions would be to lessen the burden on Alberta's hospital system by picking workers' compensation claimants out of the queue. "We're not telling anyone we're going to do it cheaper or better," said Jim Saunders, who resigned as the head of the Calgary Regional Health Authority three months after the for-profit hospital opened. "I think we're going to be price competitive [in] a very warm environment that will be exceptionally nice for the patients."[27]

Although the federal government had threatened to exercise its authority under the Canada Health Act if HRG violated the legislation, most of the pronouncements from Ottawa were ambiguous and had more bark than bite. A national election was in progress, and incumbent Liberals were anxious to demonstrate to voters that they were sincere about medicare. But when the election was over and new health minister Alan Rock was installed, the rhetoric died down considerably until, finally, the federal protector of medicare was "comfortable" with the corporation's for-profit investments in health care. Less than a week before opening, HRG met with officials of Health Canada and Alberta Health to reiterate it would obey the federal legislation.[24]

"My understanding is – although you would want to confirm it with Health Canada – that they went away comfortable that HRG was going to work within the Act," said Garth Norris, an official of Alberta Health. But Rock was not talking, hoping to maintain a low profile in the controversy in Alberta, where seniors' groups and health-care activists in the Friends of Medicare were demanding Ottawa intervene to protect the province's health system. Jim Saunders told newspapers that the federal minister had been working with "inaccurate information," but now that he'd had his eyes opened by the corporation, "there are no outstanding issues with the federal government."[28]

In fact, given Ottawa's track record during the previous ten years, it was probably fair to say that most of those involved in the federal government (outside of Health Canada, which remained ambivalent and powerless) were happy with developments in the western province. If HRG promised to attract global investors to Canada's health industry – a feat already accomplished with the support of the Sun Healthcare Group and MDS – then the company was right in line with the direction set by Industry Canada.

The opening of HRG's for-profit hospital in Calgary in the fall of

1997 set the College of Physicians and Surgeons and the provincial government on a collision course over the issue of accreditation. Initially offering cosmetic and dental surgery to Calgary day patients, HRG had no problem obtaining the necessary accreditation from the College, responsible for regulating surgical clinics. But when HRG applied to expand its services to include procedures that would require patients to stay overnight, the College said such stays would change the status of the facility to a hospital, and only the province could regulate hospitals. According to the government, the legal definition of a hospital in Alberta was a facility that was publicly funded, and therefore the College did have authority to regulate HRG. The health minister, Halvar Jonson, "has taken the football and thrown it over here," said Carol Kraychy, a lay member of the college council. "But we know how to throw it back," she told a meeting of the council, adding that "this is only the first of many applications that are going to be coming down the pike."[29]

The tangle with the College convinced HRG that it did not, after all, want to be classified as a hospital but rather as a "surgical corporation." The Klein government responded swiftly, saying that HRG was not a hospital, but a "clinic," a move that put the facility back into the jurisdiction of the college. So what was the difference? Not much, according to the United Nurses of Alberta (UNA). A UNA comparison between HRG and the now closed Grace Hospital showed that the services on the menu at HRG (which had simply taken over the former Grace) bore a remarkable similarity to those once available at the hospital. Each offered (or had offered) 24-hour care, three operating theatres, rehab services, day surgery beds, recovery facilities, X-ray and diagnostic services. The Grace was defined as a hospital. HRG was defined as a clinic. Heather Smith, head of the UNA, said the provincial government's designation of HRG as a clinic "is obviously an attempt to circumvent the requirements of the Canada Health Act."[30]

HRG officials had a well-rehearsed response to critics who said the for-profit hospital spelled the end of medicare in Alberta. Dr. Steve Miller, chief medical officer of HRG, said the facility would not take away anything from the public system. Miller, like other surgeons practising at HRG, promised he would only work part time in publicly supported hospitals – although none of them would be in Calgary's inner city because all had been closed by the province. Since his public waiting list for bone surgery was six months long, he said, HRG would enable him to alleviate the problem by providing surgical services for the Workers Compensation Board and other third-party payers. But Wendy Armstrong, executive coordinator of the Consumers' Association of Canada in Alberta, said her group was opposed to the licensing of HRG. "The international body of evidence shows that what they are going to do is drive up the cost of health care and reduce access in the public system," she said.[31]

In December 1997 the College rejected HRG's bid to open overnight beds in Calgary by a vote of 17 to 1. Instead, the College demanded that the province initiate a public debate about public and private health care and "the slippery slope of two-tier medicine" that was emerging because companies like HRG wanted to compete with publicly funded nonprofit hospitals. "This is an issue that is bigger than the College," said registrar Larry Ohlhauser, "it's bigger than our profession." University of Alberta health economist Dr. Richard Plain said the decision of the College left the door open to two options: either HRG could convince the province to declare its facility a public hospital, or the province could change the law to allow HRG to operate as a full-fledged, for-profit hospital. Plain said if the province chose the first option, HRG would have to be publicly administered, something that would defeat the whole purpose of setting up a for-profit hospital in the first place.[32]

The Klein government, faced with mounting opposition to HRG, declined to grant the company approval for overnight stays. Jim Saunders, HRG's president, said the company would have to "regroup." "We will look at our options," he said, adding HRG would have to work harder to get its message across to a public that feared Americanization of the health-care system. During the spring of 1998, the province tabled amendments to the Hospitals Act that would allow the Minister of Health to grant approval to private companies that wanted to operate outside the publicly funded health system. The government also introduced amendments that would require the College of Physicians and Surgeons "to regulate the quality of patient care," including care offered in private for-profit facilities.

If the experience of Americans is anything to go by – and it increasingly is – the fight against for-profit hospitals in Canada is just beginning. The campaign mounted by Alberta's Friends of Medicare against HRG continues, and it is one that all Canadians can learn from. It is a fight that has shed light on the strategies pursued by employers, insurers, and for-profit health companies as well as by politicians who favour a larger role for the corporate sector. The fight underscores the centrality of the workers' compensation system in the expansion plans of health and insurance companies. The partnership between the corporate health sector and employers reinforces a focus that both groups have on control – control of data, demand, disability, utilization, treatment protocols and physician practices, integration, early return-to-work, workers, and providers. It is an obsession that formed a central theme in the private managed care revolution reshaping the entire health industry in North America during the early 1990s. In Canada, the workers' compensation system is providing an open window through which the private insurance industry, in partnership with employers and for-profit companies, can introduce what they term "American innovations" without violating the Canada Health Act. And it is a window through which the rest of the health system can easily be pulled.

TEN

Dealing Drugs
in Canada

Employers were experiencing some success in their efforts to control the behaviour of their employees, but their attempts to influence the pharmaceutical industry were not similarly rewarded. Drugs were acknowledged to be the biggest cost driver on supplementary benefits plans and employers were complaining that the early discharge strategies being implemented by hospitals, where drugs were covered by public plans, had led to a further shift of costs to business. Their assertions were supported by studies indicating that between 70 percent and 80 percent of all claims submitted to private plans in 1994 were related to drug purchases. Coupled with hospital early-release policies, however, were developments in the public policy arena that were sending drug prices into an upward spiral.

In 1987 the multinational drug industry got a major boost when the Mulroney government enacted Bill C-22. The legislation weakened the country's ability to control drug costs using a licensing arrangement that allowed cheaper, Canadian-made, generic – or copy-cat – drugs to reach the market before brand-name patents expired. Despite denials by Ottawa, it was widely acknowledged among trade experts (and reported in U.S. newspapers) that passage of C-22 was necessary to win Washington's approval of the Canada-U.S. Free Trade Agreement.

In 1993, on the eve of signing the North American Free Trade Agreement (NAFTA) with the United States and Mexico, Canada enacted Bill C-91, granting twenty-year patent protection to expensive, brand-name drugs, most of which were manufactured and distributed by the powerful U.S.-based pharmaceutical industry. In what was seen as a major victory for U.S. drug firms, extended patent protection was written into the trade deal in spite of Canada's boasts that it had secured protections for the health-care sector. By early 1997, Bill C-91 was undergoing a mandatory review by a parliamentary committee amidst a wave of criticism. Prime Minister Jean Chretien pleaded with an angry public for understanding: the government, he said, was "compelled" by the two trade deals to extend the lengthy patent protection for brand-name pharmaceuticals, "unless an epidemic broke out or something like that."[1]

Bill C-91's deregulation of the drug industry led to spectacular increases in the cost of drugs, costs that Canada could once point to as the lowest in the industrialized world. From 1987 to 1996 the cost of prescription drugs in Canada rose by 93 percent, compared to an increase in the Consumer Price Index of 23.1 percent. Drug costs grew proportionately faster than any other item on the nation's health bill, from 9 percent of total health expenditures in 1984 to 12.7 percent in 1994 and over 14 percent two years later. Spending on hospitals and physicians, meanwhile, decreased from 42 percent to 37.3 percent of total health expenditures, and from 15 percent to 14.2 percent, respectively. At the same time, Canada ranked at the bottom (along with the United States) of the OECD's list of twenty-four countries that made publicly insured drug plans available to its citizens. Only 43 percent of the population was eligible for coverage on provincial pharmacare programs, and those who were eligible often paid prohibitively high deductibles on drug purchases. As drug prices continued to rise, workers sought relief in employer-sponsored benefits plans.[2]

In 1994, US$256 billion was spent on prescription pharmaceuticals around the world, and annual sales grew by between 10 and 16 percent in each of the next three years. Today North America, Western

Europe, and Japan together account for about 80 percent of world drug purchases in a market dominated by U.S. and European brand-name products. Drug companies are expanding rapidly into developing countries and the new markets of Eastern Europe – where preferences for natural and dietary remedies are referred to as a "cultural barrier" by the industry. Many drug makers are entering the "alternative drug therapy" business. Among Eli Lilly's twenty collaborative ventures, for example, is a deal with Shaman Pharmaceuticals Inc., a company that combs the world's rain forests in search of so-called folk remedies. "They take the plants found by medicine men or witch doctors and try to identify what is the active ingredient," said Lilly's research chief Dr. August Watanabe. He did not mention that once the "active ingredients" were identified, they likely would be patented by Lilly and Shaman, requiring the "medicine men and witch doctors" to submit a royalty fee to the corporations next time they prepared a folk remedy.[3]

Patented drugs and generics

Canada's drug industry is relatively small, composed of 119 companies that produce or distribute pharmaceutical products. Eight of the top ten companies with over $100 million in 1996 annual sales are foreign-owned, brand-name pharmaceutical corporations. Foreign multinational drug companies accounted for 87 percent of drug sales revenue, but 63 percent of all prescriptions filled. Generic Canadian brands made up only 13 percent of sales revenue and 37 percent of prescriptions filled in Canada. The higher percentage of revenues relative to market share is one way of illustrating a well-known fact of life in the drug business: brand-name pharmaceuticals are more – much more – expensive.[4]

Profits among the ten leading U.S. drug makers totalled US$18.6 billion in 1995 on sales of US$106.2 billion. During the 1990s, mergers have reshaped the U.S. industry and, by extension, have changed Canada's drug market, which is dominated by U.S.-owned companies. In 1996, merger and acquisition deals in the drug industry were worth US$41.2 billion, up from 1994's record US$36.1 billion. Obviously acquisitions cost money, spurring further increases in drug prices so that acquiring companies need not gouge their profit margins to offset the amounts spent on expansion. These price increases have occurred in spite of the efforts by managed care companies, U.S. federal and state politicians, employers, and consumers to rein in the cost of drugs.[5]

As cost increases spilled over into Canada, provinces responded by increasing deductibles for public plans and introducing more stringent eligibility criteria. They also delisted drugs from public plans or implemented rules that required patients to purchase cheaper, and sometimes less-effective, brands. As payments for delisted drugs shifted to health plans sponsored by employers groaning about escalating premiums, drugs became a target of cost-conscious benefits managers who began negotiating bulk discounts with manufacturers of cheaper, often generic alternatives. In response, the pharmaceutical giants embarked on a costly spending spree to plug what was seen as a potential threat to their profits.

The drug industry has added an array of new terms to the health-care dictionary during the last fifteen years. Pharmacy benefits managers (PBMs), for example, were insurers who sold claims adjudication services to employers and insurers. PBMs were arbitrators who adjudicated, or passed judgment on, the insurance claims submitted by employees who wanted reimbursement for their drug purchases. PBMs relied heavily on information technology, which enabled them to electronically monitor and process claims and provide employers and insurers with details of each employee's prescription drug patterns. The PBM would draw up what was referred to as a "formulary," a basket of insured drug options, and doctors were required to prescribe only those drugs included on the plan. If a patient chose a drug not included in a PBM's formulary, the patient would have to pay for the prescription instead of the insurer. With drug costs rising, insurers and plan sponsors placed mounting pressure on PBMs to put cheaper generic brands in the drug basket.

In the early 1990s many U.S. drug makers merged with pharmacy benefit managers that administered prescription drug claims for managed care health plans. These mergers allowed manufacturers to exert control over which drugs in the PBM's formulary were given preference and to influence the choice of prescribing physicians. But it was a strategy that cost the pharmaceuticals a pretty penny. In 1993, Dupont Merck acquired Medco Containment Services for US$6.6 billion, while London-based SmithKline Beecham paid US$5.2 billion for a U.S. drug benefits company. A year later Eli Lilly bought PCS Health Systems Inc. for US$4 billion, bringing the total of the three buyouts close to US$16 billion, a hefty price to pay for a foothold in one of the fastest-growing sectors of the U.S. health industry.[6]

Many of the insurers and employers who paid the spiralling drug bills viewed the entry of the big brand-name companies into the PBM field with relief, expecting a managed care approach to lower their drug costs. PCS and Medco together managed pharmacy benefits for 80 million Americans and had gained favour among corporations and HMOs looking for someone to process prescriptions claims, monitor physician prescribing practices, and negotiate volume discounts with pharmaceutical companies.

But the U.S. Federal Trade Commission (FTC) was alarmed. When the two drug benefits managers were sold to Merck and Eli Lilly, the FTC warned the companies that they could face anti-trust charges if their new acquisitions gave preferential coverage to the parent company's brand of drug. It was not the FTC's job to protect patients from rising drug prices or from corporate strategies that led to astounding increases in drug-company profits. Its job was to create a level playing field for competing companies. Thus in the mid-1990s the Pfizer Corporation's successful suit against Lilly, which ensured that its cheaper anti-depressant Zoloft was getting treatment equal to Lilly's Prozac from Lilly subsidiary PCS, was testimony to how well federal regulations were working. Unfortunately, the court's ruling did not result in lower overall drug costs for American consumers.[7]

In Canada, prices on patented drugs – which make up about 45 percent of the market – are regulated by the federal government's Patented Medicine Prices Review Board (PMPRB), while nonpatented drug prices are regulated by the provinces. Created in 1987, largely in response to the negative reaction to Ottawa's patent legislation, the PMPRB's job is to ensure the prices charged by manufacturers of patented drugs are not excessive. But the board has not succeeded in this mission. Since it was established, the PMPRB has allowed the cost of medicine to increase annually by a whopping $3 billion, undoubtedly because the drug companies supply the data used by the board to determine "fair prices." This fact became the focus of criticism by Opposition MPs and the Canadian Health Coalition, a group of health activists, during the federal government's review of Bill C-91 in early 1997. These critics were joined by former staff and members of the board who charged that domestic drug prices were based on inflated figures that in many cases were double what consumers paid in the United States and Europe. The drug industry argued the rise in drug costs was due to increased use by Canadians, not increased prices. This argument was ultimately accepted by the federal government despite the mountains of contrary evidence.[8]

The main benefactors of the new drug regime were the foreign-owned, brand-name pharmaceutical companies, which stepped up their sales and marketing activities in Canada after the patent legislation was passed. In response to corporate concerns about escalating drug costs and both public and private drug plans' growing preference for cheaper, generic alternatives, pharmaceutical companies began importing the techniques they had successfully employed in the U.S. managed care market.

Managed drug care

In 1994 Merck and Lilly, noting that PBMs were nonexistent north of the border, said they hoped their benefits management idea could be adapted to markets outside of the U.S. Less than a year later, Lilly Canada announced it had taken a "bold step into Canadian managed health care" with the acquisition of Sudbury-based RXPlus, a company that managed health (as opposed to pharmaceutical) benefits for 500,000 employees on employer-sponsored plans and that was "poised for aggressive growth and rapid expansion" of its customer base. Describing the "marriage" as a "uniquely Canadian initiative [designed] to fit the Canadian health care context," Lilly Canada President Nelson Sims said the purchase of RXPlus would help "kick-start" managed care in Canada. He vowed to "always put the customer's interest first." The customer in this case, of course, was the employer who contracted with RXPlus, not the employee.

But the deal was raising eyebrows in a number of quarters across the country, not least in Canada's generic drug industry. "Isn't there a potential conflict of interest when Lilly appears to be in a position to influence which drugs appear on RXPlus's formulary?" worried observers asked. "Is it ethical for a drug manufacturer to own a drug claims adjudicator?"[9]

While benefits consultants pondered these questions, Sims was busy dismissing their concerns. "Our approach is that [the conflict of interest charge] is a non-issue," he said. Lilly had met with Canada's competition board before and after the sale of RXPlus and no objections had been raised. But even some Liberal MPs were worried. Dan McTeague, a Liberal MP from Ontario (who apologetically asserted that Ottawa was "napping" when the sale of RXPlus took place), warned "the risk of conflict is there." Drug companies "who are hard pressed to increase earnings on a broader scale now have third-party adjudicators who can influence large benefits plans," he said, adding that "you can't help but be suspicious and alarmed."[10]

But the most outspoken critics were Canada's generic drug makers, who demanded the federal government overturn the deal. "This is a dangerous mixing of manufacturers and prescribers," said Jim Keon of the Canadian Drug Manufacturers' Association (CDMA), the group representing generic drug companies. The acquisition, the CDMA said, "could foreshadow similar buy outs of other Canadian pharmacy benefits companies by brand-name drug manufacturers, as has occurred in the United States." And they were right. By the end of 1995 Medco said it wanted a share of the Canadian market too, and rumours started to swirled that the company would soon be north of the border.[11]

Amidst charges that "this industry incest has a decided made-in-America look about it," employers maintained a vigilant silence on the acquisition. They were responsible for the 20 percent increase over one year in the number of employees covered by the Lilly RXPlus plan. Lilly's sales pitch for its managed care package included a magnetic "smart card" issued to each employee that was used whenever a prescription was filled. If the drug being purchased was not encoded on the card, the pharmacist would know the employee must pay. If the RXPlus card gave the pharmacist a green light, the claim would be processed and paid for by the insurer in a matter of seconds. Critics charged that smart card technology would lead to increased drug use, in part because it encouraged more frequent drug purchases, a pattern that was well established in the U.S. market. Employers argued they would benefit by gaining information on employees' drug use, which would make its way into a data bank for use by the boss. But more importantly for Lilly, profits from smart card technology had increased in the U.S., and that was the plan for Canada, as well. For employees and their families, the smart card was another loss of autonomy and control over a vital aspect of their lives.[12]

Some in the benefits consulting business predicted increases in insurance premiums of between 15 percent and 30 percent "over the long haul" to help pay for increased drug use by employees covered by employer-sponsored plans and for the acquisition of PBMs by pharmaceutical companies. It was a prediction taken seriously by the insurance industry. In 1995 three leading insurers in the Canadian market – Manulife, Aetna, and Prudential – announced they had recently signed agreements with a St. Louis-based PBM, Express Scripts, Inc., to manage their clients' drug benefits and "provide detailed reports to employers" on employee drug use. Since drug claims would be processed electronically in the United States, the companies would need a "data processing exemption" from the federal government so they could send patient information over the border and verify they intended to "keep control of the data and protect privacy." Other insurers – Sun Life, Great-West Life, Canada Life, and Mutual Life – already had a joint ownership arrangement with the Winnipeg Simkin family in Shared Health Management of Ontario, the largest electronic benefits manager in the country.[13]

The price of drugs in Canada helped boost the excessive profits earned by the industry worldwide. Pharmaceutical companies asserted that drug industry profits, more than three times the median for all 500 industries in *Fortune* magazine's annual tabulation, were required to offset the risks involved in research to develop new, more effective medicines. But of eighty-one new patented drugs introduced in Canada in 1995, only two were defined as "breakthroughs," compared to three out of sixty-four the previous year. Drug companies also claimed that Canadians had benefitted from the creation of nearly 5000 new jobs in the industry since 1987, a figure contradicted by Statistics Canada, which reported a decline of 1500 jobs between 1991 and 1995. "The facts speak for themselves," the Pharmaceutical Manufacturers' Association of Canada said in an advertising blitz during the Bill C-91 review. While Canadians fumed about twenty-year drug patents and deregulation, the multinational drug industry, claiming the federal review board was doing an "outstanding" job, praised Ottawa's "world-class patent protection," which "has been good for Canada and Canadians."[14]

The entry of pharmacy benefits managers into North America's health industry did not bring about reductions in the cost of drugs nor the "savings" PBMs promised they could achieve by negotiating bulk discounts with pharmaceutical companies. Instead, the pharmaceutical industry posted record profits, and drugs consumed a larger and larger portion of Canada's total health expenditure. The burden on employer-sponsored health plans was sending businesses into a frenzy, but it was a burden felt in the hospital sector as well, which needed drug regulation, not PBMs, to control rapidly escalating costs. Most provincial and federal governments preferred to leave management of the drug market to private interests whose objectives were contrary to what the health sector needed and what the Canadian people wanted. In short order there were new companies taking advantage of the opportunities created for them in drug and "disease management."

Late in 1997, as doubts about the cost-effectiveness of managed care were mounting among employers and benefits managers in the United States, Eli Lilly announced it was moving away from "the managed health care area." RXPlus was on the chopping block, sold to an unnamed group of private health-care investors in Toronto. Michelle Noble, manager of corporate communications at Eli Lilly, said the sale of RXPlus was a "strategic business decision by Lilly to focus on our core pharmaceutical business." That business included marketing strategies that partnered the drug company with patient groups, such as the Canadian Diabetes Association, to help their members manage their chronic diseases. Disease management was in, and managed care was out.[15]

Managing 'disease states'

"Disease state management" (DSM) is a product of the pharmaceutical industry, vigorously promoted as a new science based on intensive drug therapy and seen as a cheaper and more cost-efficient approach than expensive hospitalization. It is a strategy that involves collaboration between physicians, hospitals, insurers, drug companies, and employers to manage chronic conditions such as diabetes, asthma, and hemophilia. The primary goal of DSM is to increase corporate profits by reducing patients' use of health-care services and modifying their behaviour so they will use what are referred to as noninstitutional alternatives, such as drugs.

Searle Canada, a pharmaceutical subsidiary of giant U.S. chemical manufacturer Monsanto, Inc., has developed a disease management strategy that employs managed care techniques, partnerships, and information systems on a large scale. David Caspari, a Searle official, described the "forces driving change" in North America's health-care industry to a conference in 1997. The increased demands of the "boomer bulge," he said, promise to enhance pharmaceutical sales, but this is countered by the threat to drug company profits posed by cost-cutting governments and institutions. Similarly, the development of clinical practice guidelines that determine how patients will be treated could present problems unless drug companies jump into the picture to ensure their products are part of the recommended therapy. And finally, the devolution of responsibility for health from federal and provincial governments to regional or community-based authorities and to employers has created uncertainty about who will be making the critical decisions about patient care in future. Drug companies, Caspari said, were looking for "a larger piece of health care spending" within this shifting environment. Inspired by the managed care movement in the United States, Searle was beginning to promote DSM in Canada as a solution to the panic caused by the revenue squeeze.[16]

In order to manage diseases, DSM depends on information collected by physicians who treat chronic patients and have what Searle refers to as "disease knowledge." DSM promoters sponsor Internet websites, developed in partnership with patient support groups, and collaborate with the pharmaceutical industry to develop and market standard of care guidelines. In November 1996 Searle scored its first Canadian success when it launched the Arthritis Canada Website, a partnership with the Arthritis Society and the Canadian Rheumatology Association. It was a model of "a public and private partnership, and the direct involvement of knowledgeable professionals," said John Manley, the federal minister of industry who helped unveil the site. The site would provide patients with "direct access and informative health-related information" and would also include a "private area where [rheumatologists] can interact." Searle, which provided an educational grant to the project, accepted the gratitude of its new partners. "As part of our commitment to total patient management," said the company's Canadian general manager, Chris Nelson, "[we have] placed an emphasis on developing new and innovative patient education tools such as Arthritis Canada." The website, which provides some useful information about the disease, medications, and treatment, also offers a direct link to Searle Canada where patients can deposit their names and addresses in the corporation's data bank.

Only the naive or the dishonest maintain that drug companies are developing relationships with patients and patient groups to provide empowering information. Like many pharmaceutical companies, Searle has colonized specific chronic conditions and its educational efforts, not coincidentally, complement its role as a leading supplier of arthritis drugs. Other companies also are affiliated with support groups representing patients to whom they sell drugs and supplies. For example, Eli Lilly, the corporate affiliate of the Canadian Diabetes Association, also produces insulin and provides diabetes education at $195 for a three-hour session. Lilly posters decorate the walls in diabetes centres located in hospitals across the country, informing patients of the company's selfless contribution to diabetes management and research. Thomas Trainer, Eli Lilly's chief information officer, says the company offers "an information product wrapped around a pharmaceutical product," and has identified educational videos and customer quizzes as effective marketing tools.[17]

Searle and its strategic partners also place patient education within the context of a broader agenda than simply producing informed customers. "Why is the Pharma industry moving into DSM and managed care?" Caspari asked conference attendees rhetorically. His answer: the marriage of DSM and managed care promises new opportunities – or new centres of profit – for the drug industry. DSM gives pharmaceutical companies like Searle access to "disease-specific data" (i.e., patient information) and to new markets for its services and products. In addition, DSM has the potential to enhance the drug company's corporate image, lending it a competitive edge and providing a platform to influence "guideline development" and standards of care.

Searle's partners in these endeavours include other drug companies with capital and valuable links to the medical profession, patients, and government. Academics provide Searle with the clinical expertise needed to develop practice guidelines. The insurance industry offers "actuarial science," health data, and claims management experience, while banks contribute financial resources and a large workforce made up of many people who need drugs to manage their chronic conditions. Telecommunications companies are a vital component as well, providing technology for data management and design capabilities to set up the electronic links necessary for DSM and managed care.

Searle and its partners are primarily interested in chronic patients whose incurable conditions present long-term "investment opportunities." The anticipated return on investment – or ROI – is shrewdly calculated before a single investment dollar leaves the corporate hand, despite the rhetoric about educated patients with manageable diseases. The conditions that offer the most satisfactory returns include hypertension, coronary artery disease and stroke, schizophrenia, Alzheimer's and chronic depression, the growing family of "women's health problems" (osteoporosis, fertility/infertility, menopause), arthritis, asthma, diabetes, chronic back pain, and hemophilia. The "ROI on DSM,"

Searle explains, is promising, based on secure and growing profit margins. Canadian subsidiaries provide "flow-through" value to the parent (U.S.) company in the form of disease-related data, patient information, access to patients/customers, and influence on clinical practice guidelines at the developmental stage.

If the "flow-through" to the parent company is to be realized, Canada will have to "move to a U.S.-style, HMO capitated system," said Caspari, in which the delivery of care – including decisions on what kind of care and how much – is controlled by insurers. In a capitated payment system, insurers pay physicians a set amount for each patient in their practice, regardless of how much or how little each patient uses the doctor's services in the course of a year. The HMO capitated system referred to by Caspari rewards physicians who "underutilize" or deliver less care and penalizes those who provide levels of health care that dig into the profits of the insurer. "The intent," he added, "is to be profit-generating," a challenge in Canada's mainly non-profit health-care system that rewards doctors for overutilization, or inappropriately high levels of treatment.

Another company practicing DSM techniques, U.S.-based Quantum Health Resources, was a star on Wall Street when it decided to "go public" in 1990. Quantum was known in the marketplace as a "pure play" company, because almost all of its revenues came from a single, high-tech source: home infusion therapy. This technology enables hemophiliacs to avoid repeated hospital visits to obtain infusions of a blood-clotting protein needed to control their condition. Even more alluring for pure-play investors, two thirds of Quantum's customers were hemophiliacs who used the company's home infusion equipment. As one investment banker put it, Quantum had an edge over other infusion companies that provided equipment to patients with curable illnesses. Because hemophiliacs are chronic, he said, they "represent a recurring source of revenues; you can look at it almost as an annuity." With its initial public offering, Quantum netted a handsome $27.9 million, an amount allocated to expansion and debt repayment, while investors predicted even more rewards "two or three years down the road." They were right: in 1995 Quantum was sold to the Olsten Corporation, a multinational home-care company with substantial investments in Canada.[18]

The subject of these efforts – the patient – has little to do in a DSM environment except, of course, remain chronic. Disease state management plans are not tailored to the individual patient but rather, and more importantly, are designed to trigger untapped revenue streams. DSM provides drug companies with the opportunity to collaborate with insurers and employers who may prefer to pay for prescription drugs rather than hospital or other forms of care that entail time off work (with sick or disability benefits) and more expensive but thorough treatment plans. Drug company profits remain high while employers can expect premiums to increase less rapidly and insurers enjoy lower benefit payouts. Pharmaceutical companies, tired of their portrayal as the "bad boy" in the story of spiralling health-care costs, hope to improve their public image by creating broad investment alliances and partnerships with employers, patient groups, hospitals, and physicians.

But DSM's success depends on accessing and using information contained in patient medical records and thus poses one of the most serious challenges to patient confidentiality. Increasingly, those records are stored in data banks managed by large employers or health and insurance corporations. Patients – who often must negotiate a bureaucratic maze for access to their medical charts – lack the means to track or audit the flow of information pertaining to them. This flow travels from doctor's office or pharmacy to insurers, disease state managers, and employers. But many unsuspecting patients also are submitting information about themselves on seemingly innocuous forms posted on the Internet. While patients expect to get information about a company's drug, unbeknownst to them there is a good chance that their profile will be captured in the pharmaceutical firm's data bank and used in targeted ad campaigns.

Information technology is an increasingly vital component of the worldwide drug industry, which uses the data to help it target patients in aggressive advertising campaigns. Janlori Goldman, the founder of the Health Privacy Project at Georgetown University in Washington,

D.C., got interested in the issue when she was pregnant. Suddenly she was receiving coupons for everything from children's book clubs and parenting magazines to personalized birth announcements. "Where are they getting this information?" she wondered. She never found out.[19]

Goldman worried about "the linking of doctors and health plans and drug companies" that are able to cull information about patients from "smart card" technology or from surveys voluntarily, if naively, filled out by patients. Statistics about gender, age, income, educational status, and health conditions – everything from what kind of allergies individuals have to how they treat yeast infections – are provided by patients who have no idea how the information will be used. Information marketers provide "data mining" services, gathering health statistics from both public and private sources. Even companies like American Express, which keeps detailed information about customer spending habits (including spending on drugs and other health products), are in the business of selling that information to other companies. Information is a valuable product, and technology is the key to getting it, maintaining it, and selling it.[20]

Privacy advocates are concerned about attempts by drug companies to partner with Canadian pharmacies so they can market medicine to customers. PBMs are collecting information about patients from doctors and health-care professionals, governments, employers, hospitals, and pharmacies with few or no strings attached. PBMs and health data managers claim that the information they collect is used to help boost patient health by linking providers to one another – for a fee. Patient data already is a commodity in Canada's health-care system, travelling along an unregulated information highway. "There is nothing to [prevent] your pharmacy benefits manager from selling the fact that you got pregnancy vitamins to the diaper service company," commented one hospital clinical information officer. Little wonder that, as one commentator put it, the "mailboxes of pregnant women bulge with coupons for discount diapers."[21]

Global moguls

The drug industry is one of the most globalized sectors in an increasingly globalized health-care industry. The products manufactured by the industry can provide patients and consumers with a better quality of life and greater control over their own health. But the industry has been at the forefront of manufacturing not only drugs as a solution to ailments, but often the ailments themselves.

It also has been at the forefront of deregulation in Canada and around the world and has exerted a powerful influence in Ottawa through the Pharmaceutical Manufacturers Association of Canada, an industry trade group with a membership of mainly U.S. firms. Paul Martin, federal finance minister, has close ties with the industry as a former director of Imasco, the parent corporation of Imperial Tobacco and Shoppers Drug Mart.

In addition to exerting influence on national governments, the drug industry is active at international trade tables. Although citizens in the U.S., Mexico, and Canada were excluded from negotiations for NAFTA, the drug industry was not. It played an important role in shaping the agreement's objectives, defining its unprecedented scope and application, and ensuring the industry's interests were reflected in the final text. One group, the Intellectual Property Committee, made up of large pharmaceutical companies and other multinationals, boasted openly that its "close association with the U.S. Trade Representative and [the Department of] Commerce has permitted the IPC to shape the U.S. proposals and negotiating positions." The rules integrating North America's regulatory drug regime, or more accurately its deregulated regime, were extraordinarily influenced by the industry, much to the detriment of the people of Canada.[22]

The global drug industry is also busy mining biotechnology, an area of research that is receiving hundreds of millions of dollars for research, and is supporting partnerships with universities and hospitals. According to the federal government there has been a reduction in the number of Canadian pharmaceutical manufacturing facilities "following mergers and acquisitions and closure of some branch plants" by multinationals in the wake of free trade, which has "permitted rationalized production." With Ottawa's help, multinational firms have assigned their Canadian subsidiaries responsibility for research in specific cancers, bone disease, viral infections, and "in vitro diagnostics." The latter science involves developing genetic markers that can predict whether or not an individual is susceptible to a specific disease or will contract the disease in the future. Canadian subsidiaries also are developing products from DNA sources and from "novel animal species."

All such research is heavily subsidized by Canadian taxpayers, either directly or indirectly, through private partnerships with public research institutes, universities, and hospitals. These partnerships are a useful way for drug companies to tap into Canada's extensive medical research capability. In exchange for providing funds to a university, for example, a pharmaceutical firm not only gains access to top-notch medical researchers, but universities may also allow companies what is referred to as "right of first refusal." This is an odd way of saying that the pharmaceutical company has the right to patent new drug discoveries with a commercial potential before any other group, including the university.

Canada also has the most generous tax-credit scheme in the industrialized world for investors in biotechnology. "In Canada," the Canadian Biotechnology Strategy Taskforce said in early 1998, "the financial and policy support provided by governments have been critical to the growth of the biotechnology sector. These support mechanisms include funding basic research, assuring the supply of highly trained human resources as well as financial assistance for research infrastructure, start-ups and innovation. Government's sharing of risk is important where market entry is difficult and costly." Needless to say, the market drug companies are interested in is global. To this end, the Department of Foreign Affairs and International Trade has worked hard to boost Canadian health biotechnology companies, organizing joint trade missions to Japan, Germany, Sweden, France, the United Kingdom, and the United States over the past two years – "with good results." Government support for the biotechnology sector also is provided through drug company funding by the Medical Research Council, the National Research Council, and through five NRC institutes involved in life sciences. Technology partnerships provide another source of funding for the drug industry, while $800-million is being provided to universities, hospitals, and research institutions to improve their research infrastructure to enable them to attract drug company partners. The Business Development Bank of Canada, with a number of financial partners, finances research and development for new start-up companies. And the federal government's Export Development Corporation provides financing and insurance for the drug industry's export business. Although Ottawa cannot find money to directly support the quality and accessibility of health-care services, there seems to be an endless store of cash for the pharmaceutical and biotechnology sector.[23]

The takeover of Canadian-based companies by U.S. drug firms has increased substantially since Ottawa increased its generous financial contributions to the industry. Consequently, the demands of Canadian subsidiaries for deregulation and more money echo the voices of their U.S. parents, who have made some progress south of the border in winning lower standards for the process involved in getting a drug to market. In November 1996, for example, the U.S. government approved the use of experimental drugs on patients admitted to hospital emergency wards in an unconscious state if their lives were in jeopardy and if attempts to contact relatives were not "feasible." Supporters of the law claimed unconscious patients would benefit. Dr. Norman Fost, director of the Center for Clinical Ethics at the University of Wisconsin, who lobbied for the change, said medical research was hampered by the consent requirement. Given the choice between standard treatments and drugs that had proven successful in animal experiments, Fost said, "It seems to me that a reasonable person would very much want to be in the study."[24]

But others were not so sure. The new law came into effect when a number of U.S. physicians were commemorating the fiftieth anniversary of the Nuremberg Code in Geneva. The U.S. law, they said, challenged a principle that dated back to the Nuremberg trials of Nazi doctors after World War II. These doctors were convicted of using human subjects in horrendous drug experiments. The Code's first principle states that no one should ever be forced to take part in a medical experiment. "The voluntary consent of the human subject is essential," the Nuremberg judges wrote. Obviously they had not foreseen the day that consent would be seen as a barrier to getting drugs onto the market. "1996 is the fiftieth anniversary of Nuremberg," said Georgetown University bioethicist Robert Veatch. "In the United States, we are commemorating that event by adopting regulations that flat-out are in violation of the Nuremberg code."[25]

Canada, too, is relaxing its drug review process. Despite the increasing complexity of drugs that result from research in biotechnology, the industry is demanding – and getting – substantial reductions in the time required to investigate whether or not new products are safe and whether they achieve the results the manufacturer claims. In 1998 Ottawa bragged that it had reduced the review time for new drugs from an average of 38 months in 1994 to 19.5 months in 1995 and to just 18 months in 1997.[26]

In 1997 there were 224 biotechnology firms, with combined revenues of about $1.1 billion. The sector received over $1 billion in venture capital funding from the growing list of investors attracted to the industry. Approximately 60 percent of the biotech firms focus on health care and thus are designated as "biopharmaceuticals," a sector that employed 4000 Canadians in 1996. Some of the largest biopharmaceutical firms are BioChem Pharma based in Montreal; Allelix Biopharmaceuticals, a subsidiary of giant MDS Inc.; QLT Photo Therapeutics; and Winnipeg-based Cangene, a subsidiary of Apotex.

Contract research organizations (CROs), which undertake clinical trials for the drug industry, are a booming sector in Canada. The Canadian government is working hard to promote the country as an ideal site for clinical trials by promoting the use of Canadian patients in drug testing programs for multinational pharmaceutical firms. Many insurance companies in the United States have declined to insure patients participating in clinical trials, as the outcomes and the consequences are unpredictable. But with Canada's universal medicare program, drug companies need not worry that a lack of insurance coverage will dampen patients' enthusiasm for participating in drug experiments. MDS, Canada's largest health corporation, is also one of the world's largest CROs and, along with its pharmaceutical customers, is pushing for quicker turnaround times in the drug approval process. The focus of the federal government has shifted from health protection to the issue of how to "focus and concentrate ... efforts to optimize commercial returns and reinforce industrial growth." Canada's regulatory review process must be "effective and efficient ... if we want to maintain and attract contract research and clinical trials work to Canada." Timely review of new biodrug products, says Ottawa, "is important, because 'first to market' is often a critical success factor."[27]

The pharmaceutical industry is in need of regulation, and drug prices are in need of an overhaul. The solutions proposed during the early 1960s by the Royal Commission on Health Services are still relevant today, including recommendations that would have instituted bulk purchasing at national and provincial levels, public ownership of pharmaceutical discoveries that occur in universities or hospitals, and the rejection of a patent system that gives manufacturers a long-term monopoly on drug products. Canadians also need protection from pharmaceutical firms that use information about their health and drug use and that sell this information to other companies. In addition, Canadians are in great need of regulations that will protect them in the future from becoming guinea pigs in experiments – with or without their consent.

But the Canadian government is moving in the opposite direction, a direction that promises to drain the health system of funds needed for longer-term health-care solutions and patient education. "Canadian biopharmaceutical research is world class," Ottawa boasts, but at the same time the country's nonprofit health-care system is in danger of being left behind in a world dominated by market medicine, and Canadian patients are in danger of being sacrificed to the interests of a drug industry with few ethics and a voracious appetite.

ELEVEN

Traffic On the Information Highway

Drug firms are not the only corporations interested in health information. The worldwide market for information technology – that is, the buying and selling of high-tech equipment, software, and support services – has an estimated worth of $3 trillion. But that total doesn't include the value of goods and services that travel the information highway. Information is itself a commodity because, like labour, it adds value to other goods and services, enhancing the profit margins of companies that market information as a raw material, as well as those companies that apply it to their own products.

Health information is one such profit-enhancing commodity. It has enormous potential to strengthen people's autonomy and control over their own health, improve the quality of services in the publicly funded health system, and greatly strengthen the values that make that system universally accessible and affordable. Within the current policy framework, however, health information is merely another consumer good bought and sold in the marketplace.

The information highway has an illusory character, but it is made up of easily understood components. The gateway, or on-ramp, is hardware – sophisticated equipment sold by large global electronics giants like IBM, Hewlett-Packard, Intel, Toshiba, and Siemens. The apparatus is expensive but vital; without it one goes nowhere. The manufacture of these implements requires access to resources (for example, water, silicon and quartz), skilled designers and engineers, and "knowledge workers." Corporations have globalized the high-tech assembly line to exploit tax incentives; skilled, low-paid labour in countries such as Malaysia and India; and guarantees that governments will lower labour standards or curtail the organizing activities of unions. High-tech hardware isn't a field for the small and modestly endowed company with limited capital and resources; even large multinationals are forming strategic alliances with their competitors to share the high costs and risks involved in developing successive waves of ever more sophisticated technology with ever greater memory capability.

Once through the gate, information is transported through a telecommunications network supplied by corporations such as the Bells, AT&T, MCI, and Northern Telecom. Provincial phone companies in Canada are forming alliances with electronics corporations to combine their products into integrated, marketable packages of hardware, software, and applications (this last is better described as how information is used and to what end). Corporations developing applications for health information cover a broad range. SmartHealth (owned by the Royal Bank of Canada and Texas-based EDS), IMS (a partnership between IBM and several provincial phone companies), and Health-Streams (formerly part of U.S. FoxMeyer's empire), CareLink, MDS, and HBO & Company are among many names and acronyms that dot the landscape in the health applications business. The applications they develop track patient records through the system from physician's office, hospital, physiotherapy clinic, or pharmacy to insurer, employer, drug firm, private lab, or nursing home company.

The third component on the information highway is information itself. Patient medical records provide valuable intelligence to pharmaceutical corporations developing strategies to market their drugs, to employers preparing to curb employees' use of health-benefits plans, or to insurance companies introducing managed care and higher premiums. Not surprisingly, therefore, gathering information about the patterns of drug use in any given community, details about when and why employees book off sick, or information that enables insurers to manage the use of the health-care system as a whole is a lucrative and highly profitable endeavour.

CANARIE on the 'Health Iway'

The physical components and public policy framework of Canada's health information highway are under construction. Despite its incomplete structure and inadequate regulatory framework, the country's information technology and telecommunications (IT&T) industry has already mushroomed, with over 400,000 employees across the country and annual revenues of $65 billion. The federal government is committed to help in a variety of ways, such as extending generous financial support and creating the necessary political and regulatory environment for corporations doing business in the sector. Provincial governments are competing with one another to attract investment to the health IT&T sector, offering tax incentives, facilitating partnerships between hospitals and corporations, and offering lucrative contracts to companies to manage public drug- and health-benefits plans. Almost all of these activities have taken place with little or no public debate or scrutiny.

The federal government has engaged in extensive consultation with the corporate sector to define the parameters of a debate that will – soon, we are told – involve the general public. Both provincial and federal governments are trying to steer a public policy course that recognizes health information as private property (thereby attracting high-tech investors) yet still protects patients as required under privacy legislation. The discussion that is taking place at this level defines health information primarily as a private good. There is no public policy debate in the media or among politicians and public officials about the benefits of prohibiting corporate ownership and control over health information altogether. Only advocates of public accountability are discussing the wisdom of vesting control exclusively in the public sector to serve both the collective and individual interests and needs of Canadians.

Ottawa is giving strong political and financial backing to the organizations developing a national information network that will integrate health-related information services and applications. "We call this infrastructure the 'Canadian Health Iway', or 'Health Iway' for short," advises CANARIE, an industry group that has identified the development of the IT&T sector as a "strategic priority" for the country. For the corporate sector this is indeed a strategic priority, however other important areas of public policy are being neglected. For example, the IT&T industry is determined to connect patients to the health system through its infrastructure of computers, telephone lines, and the Internet. This poses a challenge to the principles of universality, simply because most provinces exclude "telephone consultations" from public health-insurance plans. The issue of who pays (and how) when patients – particularly in remote and rural communities – access the health system over telephone wires has not been addressed by industry groups such as CANARIE. More to the point, the federal government's focus has been shaped by Industry Canada rather than by the federal health ministry. Thus Ottawa is primarily concerned with how to assist the industry in establishing itself in Canada, not with how to protect and enhance universal medicare.[1]

CANARIE, Inc. – the Canadian Network for the Advancement of Research, Industry and Education – is an example of how Ottawa has represented, and likely will represent in future, the many complex issues surrounding information technology in the health sector. CANARIE is an Ottawa-based nonprofit consortium of over 140 academic, business, and government organizations that was established in March 1993 as a public-private partnership between the federal government and the corporate sector. There are no patient advocates or health-care workers among the participants. These groups undoubtedly would have little to contribute to CANARIE's primary task, which is to "maximize opportunities to turn knowledge and ideas into profitable goods and services" and to create "gateways to international markets."

With strong links to Industry Canada, from whom it receives a healthy dose of funding, CANARIE was created to bring together the federal government and private sector in a collaborative effort to launch and oversee a national information highway with an emphasis on health and education. In 1993 CANARIE allocated $115 million to the first phase of its seven-year business plan. The federal government provided $26 million of the total, with a further $89 million from the private sector. By the time the group reached its second phase a year later, it had attracted another $400 million in funding and expanded its membership list to include such industry giants as Hewlett-Packard, the Royal Bank, MDS, Stentor, LARG*Net, APM, HealthLink, IBM, and Telesat Canada.

The "information highway" is not only the route to the $3 trillion global marketplace, but it is a prerequisite for what the corporate sector refers to as "integrated health care." Theoretically, integrated health delivery knits public and private providers together in a "seamless continuum" of care through which patients and their medical records move unhindered with the help of expensive information systems. A technological thread of hardware, software applications, and telecommunications connects hospitals, hospital departments, physicians, pharmacists, nurses, laboratories, and a range of health professionals. That thread – supported both financially and politically by governments and hospital administrators – increasingly leads to companies dependant on data collected by health professionals. For example, drug companies use information about the prescribing preferences of Canadian doctors and the consumption patterns of patients to develop marketing strategies. Private laboratories are better able to develop their markets when physicians are hooked up by computer, sending their lab requests and receiving results via the Internet. Suppliers can maintain fully automated "stockless distribution" systems and "just-in-time" deliveries to hospitals using a simple computer link. The possibilities are endless and public funding is available, either directly in the form of cash infusions from federal and provincial governments or indirectly in the form of lucrative contracts with hospitals and other large institutions.

Concerns about the confidentiality of patient records and information are rising specifically because of the increased involvement of private corporations in data collection and processing. Public pressure has forced both federal and provincial policy makers to address the issue of privacy and security, a responsibility of both levels of government. But current legislation at both levels is proving to be inadequate. Only in Québec are there laws and regulations applicable to both the public and private sectors. In all other jurisdictions, privacy legislation focusses on information moving among public or publicly funded providers or on safeguards against "snooping employees" in health-care institutions. But as information flows into more and more "outside" hands – both in terms of quantity and sensitivity – Canadians are becoming justifiably alarmed at how little control they have over who has access to the most confidential aspects of their lives.

It is ironic that as Canadians (like their American cousins) are advised to assume more "personal responsibility" for their health status and health care, they are losing many of the tools necessary to such an undertaking. In addition, the lack of strong regulations to protect patients' privacy and strengthen their control over access to their information has increased fears that health information will be used by banks, for example, to deny customers with a chronic condition a loan, or by employers to reject job applicants. Information technology, which has such great potential to "empower patients" with knowledge, can just as easily be used to fulfill other, less public-spirited objectives.

Info tech and FoxMeyer

As described in chapter 10, the pharmacy benefits managing industry has attracted the attention of powerful interests, notably those involved in information technology or "info tech." Drug benefits managers depend on sophisticated information collection and storage and this has led to partnerships among a range of parties including hospitals, physicians, employers, provincial ministries of health, the telecommunications and computer industries, banks, and pharmacies. These alliances, like the technology that links them, cross borders effortlessly and so, too, does the information in, which they trade. Medical information is hot, whether it is composed of treatment guidelines or patient records, and companies involved in the health-information business are thriving.

HealthStreams Technology, Inc., was one such company that billed itself as "a new and important source in Canadian health care." Founded in June 1994 as FoxMeyer Canada Inc., HealthStreams was a creature of Texas-based FoxMeyer Corporation and the Evans Health Group Ltd., a preventive health and rehab services company based in Toronto. Evans Health Group was formed in 1991 when Evans Medical Industrial Clinic merged with Canadian Neuromed Clinics. This merged company expanded four years later to include pharmacy and PBM services. The new business was operated by Gerald Shefsky, head of CST Entertainment, Inc., a company involved in digital colour enhancement of black-and-white films.

When FoxMeyer Corp. entered the picture, it brought with it a list of impressive backers well connected throughout North America. Despite the different health-care systems in the two countries, said Thomas Anderson, chairman of FoxMeyer Canada and president of the U.S. parent, advanced information technology would "enhance the effectiveness and the efficiency of delivering health care. That is FoxMeyer's mission – we are creating the North American health care business model."[2]

Within six months, FoxMeyer Canada had attracted some of the most powerful business leaders on the continent to its board of directors, not the least of whom were Canadian senator John Trevor Eyton, chairman of Brascan, deputy chairman of Edper Enterprises, and director for Norcen Energy Resources, American Barrick Resources, General Motors, London Life, Noranda, Coca Cola, and John Labatt – among other household names; Andrew Sarlos, director of Ontario Hydro, the Horsham Corporation, Alliance Communications, a member of the board of governors of the Toronto Hospital Foundation, and a founding member of the Budapest Stock Exchange; and Paul Waitzer, a former governor of the Toronto Stock Exchange and founder and CEO of Yorkton Securities. These eminent Canadians were joined by White House insiders from the United States and several members of the powerful U.S. Business Roundtable.[3]

With such prestigious connections to political and financial circles on both sides of the border, FoxMeyer Canada was ready to embark on the well-travelled road of acquisitions. "Acquisitions," a corporate report to the Ontario Securities Commission noted in mid-1997, "have played an important role in the creation of FoxMeyer Canada. We continue to believe that the health care delivery system throughout North America is fragmented, and that vertical and horizontal integration of synergistic businesses can provide long-term value to shareholders."

The company pursued this credo with zest. After a buying spree that strengthened its foothold in central Canada, FoxMeyer was rewarded with a contract from the Québec government to electronically process drug claims for the province's senior citizens and welfare recipients, linking 1400 pharmacies to the provincial drug-benefits management program. Later that year the Ontario Public School Boards' Association, with 250,000 employees across the province, signed an agreement with FoxMeyer to manage its pharmacy benefits plan, one of the largest such contracts ever signed in Canada.[4]

But FoxMeyer had other strategies to establish its business model in the Canadian health-care marketplace and thereby "grow" its business. The purchase of Québec-based Medisolutions in April 1996 gave FoxMeyer the critical mass it needed to extend its "information technology solutions to all providers in the health care delivery system" in Canada, and most importantly in the "growing Hospital Information Systems segment" of the market. Medisolutions, previously known as 1st Group, Inc., brought with it 685 employees and contracts with over 400 hospitals to supply medical/administrative and software products. The company also processed payroll information for the majority of employees in Québec's hospitals and boasted over $70 million in sales revenue in 1995. The purchase of Medisolutions broadened FoxMeyer's base of hospital clients in Canada and brought "the technology behind the electronic patient record" the company needed to realize its long-term plan. With generous financial support from the Québec government, Medisolutions already had invested over $50 million in developing its product, and FoxMeyer was committed to allocating substantial resources of its own "to complete the project and market the patient medical record concept world-wide."[5]

After concluding that the PBM market in Canada was seriously underdeveloped, with less than 25 percent of employee drug claims processed electronically (compared to 80 percent in the U.S.), Fox-

Meyer jumped to capitalize "on this obvious room for growth." Its contract to provide PBM services to the Québec government was attractive but did not represent the full potential – not by a long shot. By the end of 1995 the company had established FoxCare Managed Care Network, linking 3500 drugstores across the country to FoxMeyer's data bank and giving it access to the drug-use records of thousands of individual employees. The opening of its PBM division let FoxMeyer develop contacts with major insurers and employers and market its "guaranteed savings program to encourage employers to participate in our ... PBM program." The savings program, a popular marketing tool in the U.S. health-care industry, offered nervous potential customers a guarantee that money would be saved – or the customer's fee would be less. "One of our chief goals in building this business is education of employers on the benefits of participating in the relatively new PBM concept in Canada," the company said. The lure of guaranteed savings was a good hook, and FoxMeyer was proving to be adept at reeling in the profitable catch.

But the retail pharmacy network was itself part of another, grander scheme, "the first phase of FoxMeyer Canada's community health information strategy." According to Thomas Bailey, the firm's president and CEO, the Community Health Information Network – or CHIN – "will provide the foundation to link other health care providers, including pharmacies, laboratories and hospitals, into a seamless electronic highway leading to the best possible care at the best possible prices."[6]

CHIN was FoxMeyer's model – its vision – "for the modern, efficient, integrated health care network." This network was to be a telecommunications hook-up linking health-care providers to one another and to private insurers and linking all of the above to electronic patient medical records. Among the health providers FoxMeyer would string together on the information highway were physicians, dentists, drugstores, hospitals, laboratories, insurers, and hospital and benefits administrators. Their destination was a giant – and privately controlled – repository of health-care information, a "reliable source of patient data to help maximize the cost-efficiency of health care delivery and ensure a continuum of care."

While some commentators worried that certain information-privacy issues might arise in the process of setting up such a network, it made a lot of sense – at least to FoxMeyer's shareholders – to enable pharmacists to "electronically query" a patient's doctor. Regulations protecting patients' privacy could hinder FoxMeyer's efforts, but the company said it hoped this could be overcome since "the potential benefits ... of technology applied to health care would seem to far outweigh any possible drawbacks."

One such drawback, not mentioned by the company, was the possible sale of patient information, fast becoming a lucrative market in its own right, to drug and other health-care companies who could use the data to design their marketing strategies. In exchange for collecting and managing patient information, FoxMeyer would be able to charge access fees to its long list of linked-up users – employers, doctors, hospitals, pharmacists, governments, and so on. Since any potential drawbacks were unlikely to worry Canada's friendly federal government – which was rapidly deregulating the health market – FoxMeyer was able to concentrate on its efforts to develop these "synergistic relationships" and to connect pharmacies and physicians' offices to the CHIN. As the company's Ontario Securities Commission report soberly noted, "The CHIN holds the promise of potential new sources of revenue," a point that far outweighed any privacy issues.[7]

But events in the parent company's corporate boardroom threatened to throw a monkey wrench into the plans of its Canadian subsidiary. As early as November 1995, Wall Street watchers were eyeing FoxMeyer U.S.'s long-term debt and high operating costs as well as the rising drug prices that easily outpaced the company's earnings. With what stock analysts called a "time bomb balance sheet," a heavy debt load, and plummeting income, FoxMeyer Health was in trouble. In September 1996 the company said it needed to "monetize its holdings" – or, in plain English, it was going to cash in some of its assets, including FoxMeyer Canada. In a flurry of news releases, FoxMeyer announced the sale of its Canadian subsidiary to Gordon Capital and Marleau Lemire, two investment and financial services dealers, for nearly $52 million in cash.

After the cash sale, FoxMeyer Canada changed its name to Health-Streams in an attempt to "reinvent" and distance itself from the troubled U.S. parent, two of whose subsidiaries were filing for bankruptcy. The former parent was facing a US\$198 million lawsuit by creditors who charged the company had transferred stocks and cash worth US\$450 million from its two subsidiaries just before they filed for bankruptcy. The allegedly illegal transfers, creditors said, included the stock of FoxMeyer Canada. Anticipating a legal challenge to the transfer, Gordon Capital placed the cash intended for its purchase of the Canadian subsidiary in escrow – just in case and just in time. Having survived the embarrassment of the parent's faux pas in the U.S., HealthStreams continued its charge forward on the deal-making trail, now backed and bankrolled by reputable Canadian investors. The company's board of directors said HealthStreams would soon be an "integrated managed care leader" in Canada's pharmacy benefits and hospital information systems business.[8]

Six months later, HealthStreams was "on the hunt for a partner or investor to boost its profile in hospital information systems." CIBC Wood Gundy Securities was enlisted in the search for "complementary technologies and alliances for future growth." George Czubak, HealthStreams' chief financial officer, said the company was flexible: the alliance could be in the form of a joint venture, partnership, equity investment, or acquisition. However the time was not yet right for a sale of the company. "The feeling of the board," said Czubak, "is that the full value of the share price has not been recognized as yet, and to put it up for sale would not be in the best interest of shareholders."[9]

It was reassuring to know that HealthStreams' board of directors felt such an overriding responsibility to Canada's health-care marketplace. But the questions that remained unanswered were: who has an overriding responsibility to Canadian patients? Who owns the information that HealthStreams is collecting and managing? How and why has this information become a buy-and-sell commodity?

SmartHealth and the information network

Publicly funded institutions are spending enormous amounts of money to plug in to the information age, forming partnerships with global corporations to manage health records and provide links on the health-information highway. Federal and provincial governments are spending hundreds of millions of dollars to assist in the development of privately controlled and managed patient information data banks. Both money and political commitment are required to install adequate and patient-directed safeguards on information that is now moving across borders, between providers, and among the growing legion of corporations with a financial stake in the technological revolution.

Manitoba is one province developing its high-tech industry. Besides supporting NHMC, with its robotic production facility for surgical kits described in chapter 6, in early 1996 the Manitoba government signed a deal with the Royal Bank of Canada to develop a health information network that promised to "pay off big down the line." The deal was worth $100 million to the Royal Bank, which used the money to create a new subsidiary called SmartHealth to link up all aspects of the province's health system through a computer data bank. Health Minister James McCrae said the province would save $700 million over ten years, while the opposition New Democrats said the money could have been better spent elsewhere in the health system. The Royal Bank agreed to absorb any cost overruns for its SmartHealth project, an attractive guarantee.

The health information network developed by SmartHealth promised to link doctors, hospitals, and pharmacies across the province to patient medical records detailing prescriptions received and drugs used, treatment histories, and laboratory and X-ray results. But a sizable portion of the savings projected by SmartHealth would come from the implementation of practice guidelines developed by the company that would determine which treatments would be covered under the provincial health plan, an aspect that had a number of observers worried. "Who will decide if women have to pay for Pap tests?" asked Marsha Cohen of the Institute for Clinical Evaluation in Toronto. "And will it lead to user fees?" If the treatment guidelines allowed for only one test for a diabetic with uncontrolled blood sugar levels, would the patient have to pay if further tests were deemed necessary by her doctor? However, SmartHealth won over the College of Physicians and Surgeons, which said the company had assured its members that they alone would control clinical practice guidelines – a promise that, if true, would make the province unique in North American jurisdictions that used such protocols.[10]

SmartHealth was headed by John Williams, a thirty-four-year Royal Bank veteran, who had been appointed vice president of the corporation's health industry division in 1995. His appointment reflected the Royal Bank's growing interest, and its growing investments, in the sector. In 1996 Williams was appointed a director of CANARIE, Inc., representing SmartHealth, which was seen as an important leader in "information technology solutions" in Canada.[11]

The Manitoba project presented the range of dilemmas presented to the public in the area of health information. On the one hand, the encoding of individual health records on a "smart card" had the potential of vastly improving patient care. The card would collect information whenever patients received treatment paid for by the public health plan. It meant that doctors would be readily able to access information about treatment, drugs, or hospital care received by the patient and thereby respond more quickly to illness. But on the other hand, there were many questions about whether the investment in expensive technology would net the savings predicted by the Royal Bank, savings that had not been realized in other regions where such technology was used. In addition, the collection and management of highly sensitive information by a private corporation instead of by accountable public or quasi-public bodies left patients vulnerable to the lucrative "data mining" activities encouraged by the marketplace. But very few of those involved in the debates swirling around SmartHealth in Manitoba asked why the responsibility for patient information – its collection, management, distribution, and maintenance – was given to a major bank, with a financial empire that depended heavily on customer data, instead of of deposited in the public sector.

The Manitoba government not only expected to save hundreds of millions of dollars from the new information network, but it also hoped to market the technology developed by SmartHealth across Canada, and even around the world. "Manitoba hopes to sell SmartHealth to other governments," the health minister told reporters when he announced the agreement with the Royal Bank. But before the government could sell SmartHealth, the Royal Bank sold a 51 percent stake in its subsidiary to EDS Canada Ltd., a subsidiary of Texas-based Electronic Data Systems. The "strategic alliance" would enable the two companies to "capture new opportunities in the emerging health information network market in Canada and internationally." While this left the Manitoba government out in the cold, according to Williams, the partnership would "create quality solutions in health care delivery second to none." The sale involved a commitment from EDS to invest "at least" $1 million to market Manitoba's Health Information Network (HIN) and related products across the country and world-wide. The Manitoba network "will be the first of its kind in Canada and among the first in North America," said EDS Canada's president and CEO Sheelagh Whittaker. Integrated health information networks, she said, would provide "important information on-line" to patients, health-care providers, "and the health care system as a whole."[12]

EDS, like the Royal Bank, was training its eye on the huge global health-information market. The company boasted that it "excels at collecting, organizing, and providing access to data" for health-care organizations. "The goal of these services," said an EDS spokesman, "is to link pricing and payment to treatment and outcomes," or put more plainly, to enforce practice guidelines that would cut the costs associated with procedures and services rendered by physicians and hospitals. Like the Manitoba government, physicians, too, were being pushed out into the cold, throwing the Royal Bank's vow to doctors that "guidelines are not to be drafted with intent of creating economic advantages" into doubt. Regardless of what the bank intended, EDS was now in the driver's seat and undoubtedly would bring its substantial U.S. experience to bear.[13]

That U.S. experience included a contract to maintain claims-processing software systems for the Health Care Financing Administration, responsible for Medicare. In mid-1997 the company was chosen by the Texas Health and Human Services Commission to integrate the state's eligibility criteria for health and welfare with its service delivery functions. The process, said EDS, "applies a similar kind of re-engineering of processes that transformed the banking industry some years ago," which perhaps explained its compatibility with the Royal Bank of Canada. The new system would be "tough on fraud" and computerize the state's workfare program. According to Robert Stauffer, an EDS vice president, the US$3.78 million, fifteen-month contract was "a breakthrough event," pioneering "collaborative partnerships that bring together public and private sector best practices" – the best practice, in this particular case, being methods to reduce the amount of money to assist poor people and simultaneously increase the amount going to EDS. Stauffer felt sure that the approach his company was "helping Texas develop will have the flexibility to be applied in whole or in part by other states," and undoubtedly by other provinces as well.[14]

The merger of SmartHealth and EDS may have raised eyebrows in some areas, but not among Canada's public policymakers. Industry Canada had adopted the view that by linking Canadian companies to foreign corporations it was paving the way to global health markets "where very substantial amounts of money are being spent." Therefore cross-border strategic alliances such as SmartHealth were the key to successfully developing Canada's health-information industry.

But according to the authors of a discussion paper written for Industry Canada, strategic alliances between domestic and foreign companies raise "a number of difficult, troubling problems for governments about such issues as national sovereignty ... and the control of the national economy." Troubling indeed. The authors ask, "What is the nationality of cross-border alliances? Who owns the products and process technologies developed by cross-border ... consortia?" Government control over "strategic industries such as computers or telecommunications" has been substantially eroded by cross-border alliances in these industries, "which are rapidly growing." But questions of who owns health information and on which side of the border it resides are only two among many "difficult problems" in Canada's health-information technology and telecommunications industry.

The question of whether such information should be traded and marketed as private property at all is an urgent one for Canadians, and the answer will determine how our health system functions in the future. Technology holds so much promise if it is used to enhance the fundamental values of our health system and so much danger if it allows information to become a resource mined by global corporations with goals that run contrary to the public good. It is ironic that our governments are promoting the importance of information to the health and well-being of Canadians but are keeping us in the dark about the implications of corporate control and the option of a strong public role in collecting and safeguarding patient data.

TWELVE

Outsourcing the Hospital Sector

Canada's health-care system is composed of payers, providers, and suppliers. Public payers, who in 1997 financed 68 percent of health care, are federal, provincial/territorial, and municipal governments and workers' compensation boards. Private payers – who financed the remaining 32 percent – are individual Canadians, employers, and insurance companies. Suppliers include companies that manufacture, prepare, or distribute any of a number of products from computers, surgical trays, and electricity to wheelchairs, linen, and food. Providers are institutions, companies, and individuals that organize the finances, supplies, and care that patients or clients need to stay healthy or become healthier – and they are overwhelmingly located in the private sector.

Canadian hospitals are at the heart of community health-care delivery, housing an array of clinical and support services. Although almost all Canadians believe hospitals are publicly owned, administered, and accountable institutions, the reality is somewhat different. Under provincial legislation, most hospitals – 95 percent – operate on a nonprofit basis and, in compliance with the Canada Health Act, provide publicly insured services at no extra charge to patients. But most of Canada's 850 hospitals are owned by private societies or voluntary organizations and run by community boards, voluntary organizations, or municipalities. In 1996, 87.7 percent of hospital revenues came from public payers, with the remaining 12.3 percent drawn from other sources – for example, private insurance plans and private pay patients.

Hospitals receive the largest block of provincial health expenditures, approximately 34 percent compared to almost 15 percent for physician services. Insured inpatient services include a bed and meals; nursing and other professional health services; laboratory, radiological and other diagnostic procedures; drugs; and the use of operating and obstetrical delivery rooms. The list of insured outpatient services varies from province to province, but generally includes diet counselling, lab and X-ray services, and occupational therapy, physiotherapy, and speech therapy "where available," meaning that provinces aren't penalized if such services are inaccessible. Hospitals also offer many uninsured services such as private rooms, telephones and TV sets, private-duty nursing, and cosmetic surgery, for which patients pay a fee.

In most cases, hospitals must seek prior approval from provincial ministries of health before they expand, add new programs and services, or purchase expensive technology-based systems. Once regional or provincial authorities have approved a hospital's operating budget, the facility controls the allocation of resources provided it stays within its budget and continues to provide the range of services insured by the public plan.

The remaining 5 percent of hospitals are also privately owned but operate as for-profit hospitals involved in nonacute-care services. Most long-term-care facilities or specialized services such as addiction centres are run by the for-profit hospital sector. It is not unusual for such companies to provide a certain number of beds under contract to provincial governments for publicly subsidized patients.

While provinces can – and do – influence hospitals legally (through licensing, regulations, and legislation) and financially, they are unable to actively intervene in the management and administration of individual facilities unless a government takes the extreme measure of placing hospital boards under trusteeship. This is a relatively rare step, and one that only occurs when a hospital fails to meet its financial or contractual obligations, for example, in the provision of abortion services. Thus hospitals are free, as any private corporation would be, to engage in activities with corporate partners or to contract companies to provide services.

If hospitals are privately run corporations providing publicly insured services, what does it mean to "privatize" in the hospital sector? Like services that are delisted from public health insurance, hospital services are privatized when there is a shift in who pays for those services rather than in who provides them. Often this shift occurs when administrators decide to reduce or eliminate outpatient services that are subsequently provided by businesses ready and willing to fill the resulting vacuum. The closure of outpatient physiotherapy departments across the country, for example, has led to an explosive growth in the number of rehabilitation companies whose services increasingly are paid for, in whole or in part, by private or workers' compensation insurers. The administrative decisions that cause these shifts are rarely subject to public oversight. Instead, the removal of outpatient services from the insured zone of the hospital has become a battleground between administrators facing provincial budget cuts and unionized hospital employees fighting to protect their jobs, salaries, working conditions, and, because they also are taxpayers, public health services.

Delisting from provincial health plans has been the subject of widespread attention because payment for those services moves from public to private insurers or to individuals. This is a visible form of privatization felt immediately by patients who often must pay directly for more and more necessary care. Canadians spent more than $76.6 billion on health care in 1997, a total that includes the tax dollars governments spent on their behalf for the provision of insured services, direct out-of-pocket payments, and payments made by private insurers. Of this amount, individuals spent an average of $790 each for uninsured or privately insured services, an increase of 30 percent over the average $606 they spent to purchase extra health services in 1991. Over the same period, the portion of taxes Canadians paid that went to publicly insured hospital and physician care dropped 1.6 percent, from $1761 (1991) to $1737.[1]

But these figures don't show another shift: the transfer of public health dollars from the nonprofit to the for-profit sector. It is important, therefore, to follow the money trail in the hospital sector. For while hospitals receive the greater part of their revenue from provincial governments, they increasingly act as conduits that funnel millions of public health dollars to global corporations. This transfer of public funds to the for-profit sector – a development occurring in the United States, as well – is found in a variety of arrangements, particularly in the areas of outsourcing (or contracting out), public-private partnerships, and joint ventures.

Outsourcing, integration, and core competencies

Several successive years of funding cuts have forced hospitals into an endless search for internal "efficiencies" and ways of reducing their operating costs. This has involved staff reductions, the elimination or reduction of outpatient services, the closure of some 30 percent of beds nationwide, and the reorganization or reengineering of patient care. None of these measures were enough to offset federal and provincial cutbacks. Consequently, many hospitals began grappling with questions concerning the "core mission" or "core competencies" of the acute-care sector.

According to a platoon of consultants hoping to bring their corporate clients together with publicly funded institutions, a hospital's core competency was the delivery of patient care. The core mission varied from hospital to hospital, but generally was confined to some aspect of clinical care for patients. Some hospitals, for example, that chose to develop their expertise in treating burn patients, might define that as part of their core mission. The consultants advised that though other services may be related to patient care, it was better for the hospital to focus on clinical patient care and contract out nonclinical support to companies whose core business it was to provide such services. With the helpful advice of multinational consulting firms – as opposed to the public – hospitals have begun pruning their core mission down to bare essentials, contracting outside managers to run entire departments, or outsourcing the service altogether.

The terms outsourcing and contracting out are used interchangeably with "partnership" and "alliance" and cover a variety of arrangements. Selective outsourcing is used to farm out specific jobs, for example food preparation or maintenance. Facilities management (a service captured in NAFTA) occurs when a team is hired to oversee all operations at a hospital. Transitional outsourcing brings in an "outsourcer" for a few years, after which the operations are returned in-house when the hospital has learned how to run them. And finally, full-service outsourcing turns over an entire operation, such as information systems, to outside companies. Contracting out services often displaces hospital employees, reducing the facility's labour costs while providing new opportunities for big corporations.

Most of the firms developing outsourcing as a major product line are U.S.-based multinationals whose largest source of business is often the hospital sector and whose main focus is information systems management. Marriott International (which supplies housekeeping and support services), ServiceMaster, and Aramark (support services) are all in the outsourcing business in Canada, cutting costs by paying lower wages, using part-time workers with fewer fringe benefits, and establishing broader – often worldwide – economies of scale. Hospitals also are contracting out management of whole facilities or specific departments and the provision of medical and nonmedical services within facilities. Companies may provide services such as laundry or housekeeping staff off-site, but it is not unusual for a hospital to arrange for outside managers to run its laboratory, information systems, or maintenance department directly on site. Like their counterparts in the U.S. – who outsourced about U.S.$890 million worth of services in 1995 – many Canadian hospitals have concluded that outsourcing will improve their efficiency and save money while allowing them to focus on their core mission. Information systems, housekeeping, food and management services, and equipment maintenance are the top outsourcing areas. As one hospital administrator commented, "We have world-class surgeons, but we don't necessarily make world-class meatloaf."[2]

One of the main reasons for the boom in outsourcing is that companies anticipate increased revenues and profits as hospitals, once stand-alone entities, form or join integrated delivery systems. One example of the way Canadian hospitals are integrating their operations is the move to centralized diagnostic or food services that supply several facilities in a region. Another example of this trend is the establishment of health-sciences centres that consolidate two or more hospitals under one management and financial structure. A fully integrated delivery system, or IDS, combines physician, acute care, post-acute care, outpatient services, home care, prevention, and wellness services under a single management and financial entity. IDS depends heavily on centralized planning and information systems, which are needed to track patients through the network and provide that "seamless continuum" of care. While such highly integrated networks have not been fully established in Canada, they are emerging as the pressure to pool resources and tap new streams of revenue pushes Canadian hospitals into alliances with one another and with the corporate sector.

Outsourcing has become a key component of integrated delivery systems. Many hospital administrators believe that outsourcing firms can bring greater resources and economies of scale to the tasks at hand, tasks that require enormous financial and material capacity. In an era of public funding cuts, such capacity is scarce in the hospital sector. In addition, larger companies are prepared to offer performance guarantees to build confidence and win customers in the new Canadian outsourcing market. Such contracts tie a portion of the company's fee to guarantees of savings by the hospital – if those savings aren't realized, the company's fee is decreased. This is sometimes called "risk sharing." Many contracts also guarantee a bonus to companies that exceed or improve on their original targets. This is known as "sharing the rewards."

For companies in the outsourcing business, the rewards far outweigh the risks. Global corporations that may lose a hundred or two hundred thousand dollars because they failed to meet a performance target in St. John, New Brunswick, or Toronto can easily offset the penalty with worldwide revenues worth billions of dollars a year. Performance guarantees usually do not make a noticeable dent in profit margins derived from outsourcing fees, lower wages and benefits paid to fewer employees, and lucrative supply contracts negotiated on the basis of bulk purchasing orders. Outsourcers who can provide Canada's integrating hospital sector with laundry, maintenance, housekeeping, or information technology services are poised to make a fortune.

At the London Health Sciences Centre (LHSC) and other large urban hospitals, the goal of outsourcing is to "take the work out of the operation and put that effort into direct patient care," according to a top LHSC administrator, Tony Dagnone. Refocussing the facility on its "core businesses only and divesting from non-revenue/non-core functions," Dagnone claimed in 1997, would improve the hospital's return on assets, strengthen its financial control, reduce staffing requirements, and increase its "competitive" or strategic advantage. Because of reduced provincial funding, hospitals had to compete for revenue-producing patients, introducing a fundamental market principle into the once market-free environment of the hospital sector.

LHSC, spread out over four university campuses, had already jumped into the outsourcing field with enthusiasm by the time Dagnone was spreading the gospel of competition in 1997. Service-Master Healthcare Management Services was contracted to provide integrated support services, Clintar to manage grounds maintenance, Data Business Forms to install and run the printing department with digital technology, U.S. Turbine and Laidlaw to run the energy and waste management systems, and SERCA and Summit to jointly operate the food services department. If all went well, Dagnone said, the hospital would be able to expand its market and pursue other outsourcing arrangements with the private sector.[3]

A month later, with many of the centre's operations pared down and scattered to the winds, a hospital restructuring commission appointed by the Ontario government announced that health-care services in the region would have to be consolidated. But the commission's consolidation plans did not include returning outsourced services to the health-sciences centre. Two psychiatric hospitals, LHSC's adult emergency centre, and 363 acute-care beds were slated to close, resulting in 2000 layoffs, half of them at the LHSC. Shorter hospital stays and more outpatient services in the private sector – both strategies implemented by hospitals divesting themselves of "non-revenue/non-core functions" –

allowed the steep reduction in the number of beds, said restructuring commissioner Doug Lawson. LHSC administrators agreed, saying that a facility's effectiveness could no longer be measured by how many beds it had. But others warned that bed cuts would lead to longer waiting lists and "add significant stress to an already over-taxed system."[4]

The pros and cons of contracting out

As more hospitals looked for ways to shift so-called noncore – and by implication, nonessential – functions out from under their umbrellas, a courtship was initiated by the consulting industry, which came armed with U.S. treatment protocols and reengineering designs. Cautious in the face of anticipated public opposition, consultants have viewed contracting out as a more moderate and acceptable first step towards an integrated system of health care with the full participation of the for-profit corporate sector. Consulting giants like Ernst & Young admit this is a strategy that can assist in carefully structured public relations campaigns to "educate" citizens about the virtues of the private sector and the deficiencies inherent in so-called public monopolies. The challenge for the corporate sector, Ernst & Young advises, lies first in the effective management of public perceptions, which are hostile to private-sector participation in health care, and second in changing public policies that use nonfinancial criteria – such as levels of quality, health outcomes, or universal accessibility – to measure success. To facilitate the expansion and success of private-sector involvement, a change in public policies is necessary to accommodate these interests.

But public-private deals, the consulting firm acknowledges, present some risks to Canada's health-care sector, including the risk of profit becoming "the motivating factor" instead of more heartfelt sentiments like compassion. Corporations also are known to provide many inappropriate services – for example, procedures deemed medically unnecessary by both public- and private-sector advisers – because they are profitable.

The list of potential negatives continues: extensive job loss in the public sector, threats to the confidentiality of patient information, erosion of quality care and services, negative public reaction, and increased out-of-pocket costs to consumers. Ernst & Young asserts that these risks can be minimized by effective public education, established practice guidelines, positive examples showing the coexistence of private and public systems, and clear rules governing the ownership of patient information. But none of these risk minimizers promises to improve health-care delivery. Rather they are elements of a strategy to increase public tolerance for profits for those who invest in the right companies.[5]

Health corporations assert that contracting out, or outsourcing, will achieve significant cost-savings, greater efficiency, and improved quality. These arguments hold great appeal for hospital administrators facing cuts in public funding, as well as for politicians wielding the knife, but contracting out has not been shown to be inherently better, more efficient, or less costly. "The more [health] services an entity controls," said Connie Evashwick of the Centre for Health Care Innovation in California, "the greater potential it has to save money by eliminating duplication and feeding its own services with referrals." In fact, it is rare to find global companies that contract out their support services, payroll and accounting, communications, and other components of a large enterprise because these fall outside their area of "core competency." If corporations followed the advice given to many hospitals, they would cease to exist altogether as large, diverse global firms, and the economy would be composed of numerous smaller entities each focussed on a single core mission.[6]

Nor is contracting out inherently bad; schools and hospitals would, in all likelihood, have difficulty writing and publishing textbooks or manufacturing surgical equipment. But if there are advantages to contracting out, there are disadvantages that can outweigh its benefits, including the loss of control over performance. There are often costs to the community as well, for example, the elimination of relatively well-paying, unionized jobs that provide a degree of mobility and professional career options for a largely female workforce. These costs are rarely calculated.[7]

Contracting out by hospitals presents other problems as well. While a service may be relocated from the nonprofit to the for-profit sector, the public continues to provide for its financing. Companies in the outsourcing business are consolidating rapidly across the North American continent through mergers and acquisitions and alliances. The largest companies pursuing outsourcing contracts with the hospital sector operate on a global basis, with head offices in the United States. Thus a growing number of public health dollars are following their private-sector partners across the forty-ninth parallel and into the pockets of international investors.

Are there advantages to contracting out that make the risks identified by consultants and analysts worthwhile? Commercial providers assert that they are more efficient, have lower costs, and match or exceed the level of quality in the nonprofit-hospital sector. But among more objective analysts there is no consensus. There is growing evidence that costs in the for-profit sector are, at best, the same as those of nonprofit providers, while other studies suggest that they may be even higher in the long run. In mixed publicly and privately funded health systems such as Canada's, nonprofit organizations tend to serve patients with greater care needs, more complicated diagnostic requirements, and more costly medical treatments. Since private institutions are free to pick and choose the healthiest and least costly patients, it is almost impossible to determine whether the private sector truly outperforms the public. Public and private sectors rarely play on a "level playing field," providing the same types of services to the same types of patients, so it is difficult to judge whether lower costs result from increased efficiency or decreased levels and quality of service.

Furthermore, there is no evidence supporting the claim that there is a higher quality of services in the private sector. In health care, according to one analyst, "quality is a slippery issue," and it is one that can be manipulated by businesses that adopt their own measurements to determine the "value" of services. The quality factor is becoming an important marketing tool in the United States, where escalating health costs are threatening to squeeze corporate profits in the industry. Employers and insurance companies insist that the money they spend on health services has to produce a measurable outcome. "Poor medicine and poor outcomes are bad business at any price," according to R. K. Abbott, a consultant at Watson Wyatt, a multinational consulting company. Not only are employers and insurers demanding that health-care providers offer high value and improved outcomes, but that they be able to prove it as well.

How does one measure, let alone "prove," quality of care except by the perceptions of those who use a service? Increasingly, quality measures include cost and utilization reports, disease incidence studies, and early returns to work by injured workers. Clinical evidence and medical outcomes data – something that, by definition, requires sophisticated information systems – are "tangible proof" of value and quality in health care, say a growing legion of U.S. consultants, that will force providers to "generate more effective tools for monitoring, measuring and reporting." Providers seeking accreditation in the U.S. now must upgrade their information systems in order to gather, organize, and submit data on quality – and increasingly, they are outsourcing those systems to meet the demand.[8]

If cost and quality comparisons are difficult to develop, how can Canadians know with any certainty that outsourcing will achieve the savings its promoters claim? Comparisons of costs in the United States, where the number of corporate outsourcing contracts grew by up to 46 percent from 1995 to 1996, and Canada, where the majority of hospitals continue to supply their own needs, are a good starting point. Studies comparing the two countries show that higher costs among American hospitals relate primarily to the use of more expensive non-patient-care services. Hospital support services in the U.S. (e.g., laundry and linen departments, dietary, housekeeping, equipment maintenance, and plant operations) cost 24 percent more per day than they do in comparable Canadian acute-care facilities. Overall, hospitals in Canada were 41.6 percent less expensive per discharge in 1995, with a 47.9 percent longer average length of stay. "Based on these cost comparisons," said Thomas Weil, president of Bedford Health Associates, Inc., a management consulting firm in North Carolina, "U.S. hospitals could anticipate $7.5 billion in annual savings if they reduced expenditures for support services to the levels found in similar Canadian acute care facilities."[9]

What of the savings hospitals claim they are achieving from outsourcing? Are they being used to reestablish the services that were previously eliminated, to increase salaries and wages, to rehire staff and reopen beds? The answer is no. If outsourcing is enabling some hospitals to offset years of funding reductions, this is not being reflected in expanded levels of service.

Yet despite the warnings that outsourcing should not be an organization's primary goal – "because outsourcing doesn't necessarily always save money" – many Canadian hospitals are doggedly moving in that direction, often because administrators are ideologically committed to strengthening their relationships with the corporate sector. Hospitals are undergoing a "fundamental reorganization around core competencies and strategic long-term relationships," said Michael Corbett, president of Michael Corbett & Associates in New York. "Turning to outsourcing from a cost-cutting standpoint is too short-sighted an approach," he added. "Customers should be looking to create the right kind of relationships to secure their future."[10]

One such customer was Gary Trickett, information officer at Grand River Hospital in Ontario's Kitchener-Waterloo region. In April 1996, HBO & Company, based in Atlanta, Georgia, announced it was jumping into Canada's outsourcing market, having just signed its first Canadian contract with the hospital, an acute-care and chronic-care facility. The eight-year agreement establishing a "strategic partnership" between the parties would enable HBOC to expand its Canadian presence "beyond software products to another level as a service provider." The hospital was contracting HBOC to set up and runs its information technology department, a move that, according to Trickett, would "allow [Grand River] to refocus its attention on patient care, the hospital's core business."

Founded in 1974, HBOC originally provided computer-based accounting and patient information systems to U.S. hospitals. During the 1980s the company launched an aggressive acquisition drive to position itself in the $13 billion health-information industry in the United States. Further acquisitions in the early 1990s extended HBOC's reach into the international physician, home-care, and laboratory markets. According to the company, its services and computer applications "provide the key elements for integrating and uniting providers across the continuum of care and provide the basis for a life-long patient record." With 4400 employees worldwide, HBOC markets itself as an outsourcing expert, complete with high-tech products and services for customers such as Grand River Hospital.

Trickett insisted that Grand River had conducted a "cost analysis" showing that "outsourcing was the way to go." Hospitals, he added, "are focusing on the core business of patient care and looking to establish relationships with vendors that can deliver support services more economically and with higher quality." Fourteen months after signing the outsourcing contract, Trickett became vice president of HBOC's Outsourcing Services Group, responsible for soliciting more lucrative outsourcing agreements among the nation's hospitals. He reassured the public, which probably knew nothing of the arrangement, that he would continue on a part-time basis as Grand River's chief information officer, a potential conflict of interest that received no public scrutiny by either the province or the community.[11]

Obviously outsourcing has become an important element in the integration of Canada's nonprofit hospital and for-profit corporate sectors. Despite claims to the contrary, outsourcing and other strategies to funnel tax dollars to corporations generally do not result in lower overall expenditures. In fact, Canadian statistics indicate that while provincial and federal health spending is down due to cutbacks, the amount of money spent in the private sector is increasing. And while public funding enables governments to implement health policies that meet the needs and goals of the population, as that money streams through hospitals to the private sector it becomes the private sector, not the public, that has the tools, money, and infrastructure to put policies into practice. Those policies will meet corporations' primary obligations to shareholders. A great strength of Canada's publicly funded hospital sector has been the ability of governments to exercise control over the priorities, budgets, and types of services offered by individual facilities. Increasingly, those priorities, budgets, and services are being set by international investors concerned about the rate of return on their ventures.[12]

Public-private partnerships

Hospital outsourcing and contracting out are complemented by public-private partnerships. A small army of medium-sized and multinational companies has targeted hospital board members and administrators in attempts to demonstrate the efficiency and cost savings of outsourcing and the "win-win" opportunities in public-private partnerships. But these new relationships represent a de facto integration of not-for-profit hospitals into the for-profit health industry, adapting a trend well established in the United States during the 1990s to Canadian conditions.

The conversion (to for-profit) or acquisition of nonprofit health maintenance organizations in the United States by big insurance companies during the 1990s sparked public opposition across the country as consumers saw their benefits shrinking and their insurance costs rising. But the conversion of HMOs paled in comparison to the U.S. corporate sector's aggressive assault on nonprofit hospitals. By 1997 the wave of hospital takeovers represented the largest transfer of nonprofit assets to the for-profit sector in the country's history, totalling US$9 billion in all. Today over 15 percent of the 5200 hospitals in the United States operate on a for-profit basis, and most of these are owned by a small handful of companies.[13]

As nonprofits have converted to for-profit status, the corporate sector's claims that it would improve efficiencies and lower costs have been countered by studies showing that costs have risen and services, especially for low-income earners and those requiring "charity" care, have decreased dramatically. "For-Profit Enterprise in Health Care," a landmark study by the Institute of Medicine in the late 1980s, found that when hospitals converted to for-profit ownership they boosted profits by increasing prices and soliciting business from higher-paying patients, while decreasing Medicaid and charity care. Experts who worked on the report concluded that investor-owned chains were diverting charity and lower-income patients to not-for-profit hospitals, which were forced to absorb the indigent load and raise prices to make up shortfalls.[14]

The takeover of hundreds of nonprofit or, in American parlance, charitable U.S. hospitals by health corporations was led by Tennessee-based Columbia/HCA, the world's largest health-services chain. Founded in El Paso, Texas, in 1987, with the purchase of two failing hospitals, Columbia/HCA quickly established the pattern that would catapult the company to the top of Wall Street's preferred list of health companies. To bolster its fortunes, Columbia/HCA bought a nearby competitor, closed it, and saw profits at its two original acquisitions rise. Between 1993 and 1995 Columbia/HCA purchased or entered joint partnerships with eighty-one hospitals, fifty-eight of which were non-profits. By the end of its first decade the company owned 350 hospitals, 135 outpatient surgery offices, and 200 home health-care agencies. Columbia/HCA has successfully built networks among physicians, many of whom also are investors in the corporation. These physicians have a compelling financial interest in referring patients to Columbia/HCA hospitals, whose admissions in 1995 exceeded 1.2 million.

By 1996, with 250,000 employees and annual revenues of US$25 billion, Columbia/HCA was bigger than McDonald's, bigger than General Electric – bigger, in fact, than all but a handful of other global giants. It also was the subject of a far-reaching investigation by the FBI, the Internal Revenue Service, the Department of Health and Human Services, and the criminal investigation branch of the U.S. Defense Department for allegedly defrauding and conspiring to defraud Medicare and Medicaid of billions of dollars.[15]

In 1995 Columbia decided to build a statewide, integrated health-care network in Ohio. In October the company signed its first joint venture partnership with Cleveland's nonprofit Sisters of Charity of St. Augustine Health System. It soon added a fourth nonprofit hospital to the network, St. Luke's Medical Centre, locking them into a long-term contract with Ohio Blue Cross/Blue Shield, a not-for-profit insurer. Then in 1996, Columbia/HCA became the first hospital corporation to attempt to integrate a nonprofit insurer into its operations when it announced that it would purchase Ohio's Blue Cross/Blue Shield plan for $299.5 million. The deal, said admirers of the hospital chain, would give Blue Cross "access to the capital it needs to compete in the new world of powerhouse health care alliances."[16]

The plans to purchase Ohio Blue Cross, and Columbia's aggressive assault on the state's nonprofit hospital system, instigated widespread opposition. Blue Cross customers charged that the price put on the health plan's assets was "ridiculously low" and that the nature of the transaction – a nonprofit conversion – had been misrepresented as a "joint venture." They were joined by state regulators and the attorney general in a lawsuit calling for an independent board to determine the value of Ohio Blue Cross. Adding insult to injury was the $19 million Columbia paid to the Ohio Blue Cross executives who backed the sale – leading many critics to conclude that the "platinum parachute" was, in effect, a payout to insiders to ensure the deal went through. The payouts were also questioned by the state's attorney general, who said they "were excessive and inappropriate for an organization founded to help the sick and needy."

Despite lawsuits and challenges, the pending deal got a favourable signal from health securities analysts on Wall Street, who said the sale of Ohio Blue Cross, with 1.5 million clients "in a juicy urban market," would provide "one-stop shopping," a key advantage for consumers. The acquisition would also dovetail neatly with Columbia's push to set up a network of hospitals and other health services in Ohio. But others disagreed. In March 1997, Ohio officials rejected the purchase of Blue Cross by Columbia/HCA, saying the price being paid for the nonprofit insurer was too low. Soon after nixing the deal, state regulators stepped in to take over the insurer, forbidding executives from taking any substantive actions without written consent.[17]

Columbia/HCA has been the target of organized public opposition to nonprofit conversions across the United States. The California attorney general threatened to investigate a proposed 50-50 partnership between Columbia and nonprofit Sharp Healthcare. As in Ohio, critics charged, "50-50" was actually a nonprofit conversion that would have given Columbia/HCA four hospitals and 1263 beds. While the attorney general said the deal was undervalued by between $100 million and $200 million, industry analysts approved the merger, saying Sharp was right to take less money from the hospital chain. "Columbia is a big gorilla," said Kenneth Abramowitz of Sanford C. Bernstein & Company. "In the competitive future environment you want to sell out to the strongest company you can, with the highest chance of doing well." Investment bankers warned that California's intervention, and similar actions taken against Columbia/HCA in Massachusetts and Michigan, could have a "chilling effect" on joint ventures, raising "questions of whether this 50-50 model is going to survive the scrutiny of the marketplace," not to mention of state regulators.[18]

In 1995 Columbia acquired or entered partnerships with thirty-two not-for-profit hospitals, often negotiating binding letters of intent before communities could determine whether the scheme was in their best interests. In its joint venture deals Columbia typically purchased 50 percent or more of the assets of its nonprofit partners, an arrangement that gave the corporation management control and a position from which to influence decisions to convert to for-profit status.

While Columbia/HCA was the largest and most aggressive among the for-profit chains, it was not the only one. According to Robert Kuttner, writing for the Massachusetts Medical Society in 1996, for-profit chains tend to "acquire hospitals at the lowest possible cost, invest in upgrading where necessary, close or consolidate duplicative facilities, cut staff, increase administrative efficiencies, [and] integrate vertically and horizontally." More worrying, however, was the question of whether "the for-profits ... are degrading clinical care" to maximize their returns to shareholders. In general, Kuttner said, "for-profits have ... a slightly lower overall ratio of staff to patients than non-profits," and many have been criticized for introducing inferior supplies and for replacing qualified registered and licensed practical nurses with lower paid and less trained employees. Such practices, these critics charge, deskill the health-care workforce, and because the workers receive less training from their employer, the applicability of their skills in other environments, and therefore their mobility to other jobs, is limited.[19]

For-profit companies are edging into Canada's non-profit hospital sector, too. Privately owned, financed, and operated King's Health Centre in Toronto opened in January 1996 to provide "Cadillac" health-care services to Americans. Canadians would be able to use the hospital for procedures that had been delisted by provincial govern-ments, for cosmetic surgery, and for workers' compensation services paid for by private insurers. King's banquet of forty or so services was not cheap: patients could pay up to $1595 for a five-hour medical exam that included fifteen different medical tests. "It never ceases to amaze me how much Canadians are willing to spend on their health and lifestyle if the service is right," said Ron Koval. A corporate partner in King's, Koval was also executive vice president of Banker's Acceptance Capital Corp., which specialized in medical financing and shared space in King's plush building.

King's did offer some publicly funded health-care services, but its main source of revenue was "third-party payers" – private insurers or employers who paid directly for services to get employees back to work sooner and off disability payments. It offered "new methods of disability management," Koval said, and planned to set up satellite clinics for injured workers in cities where high injury rates promised to increase business. The connection to third-party insurers was pro-vided by Ernst & Young, which helped introduce King's third-party business lines. "The basic idea," said a principal at the consulting firm, "is that the sooner a worker resumes some of his or her normal func-tions, the better for everyone. The patient gets diagnosed and hope-fully better faster, while the insurance company doesn't have to pay weeks of disability cheques waiting for test results." More importantly, the health centre and its partners all increase their profit margins.

King's investors had originally planned to open as a hospital, offer-ing "patient-pay" care with "the only available acute care private hos-pital licence in Ontario." But the province informed the company not that it couldn't operate, but rather that it couldn't bill itself as a hospi-tal because it had not been granted a licence by the Ministry of Health. When the investors got together, they decided they would operate as a "health centre" and that they therefore would not need to obtain a licence. "They did us a favour," said Scott Addision, King's senior vice president. "'Health centre' is a much more '90s title." When it opened as the legally designated King's Health Centre Corpo-ration, many of its physicians continued their regular billings to the Ontario Health Insurance Plan, turning 40 percent of their OHIP fees over to King's for overhead. The indirect OHIP funding "allowed us to start the engine of the King's Health Centre and get that critical mass in terms of revenue," said Addison.[20]

Other private companies in Canada are taking over or leasing hospital wards – or whole hospitals – to serve foreign, mainly U.S. patients. Hospital administrators looking for new revenue generators are hoping to rent space to firms such as Hospitals of Australia Corp., a subsidiary of multinational Mayne Nickless Ltd. When the company opened its Canadian division in Toronto in 1996 it said it was interested in taking over facilities in Alberta.[21]

The Australian company was interested in Alberta because the provincial government had worked hard to implement steep funding cuts and widespread hospital closures, thereby establishing the right conditions for private health-care delivery. When Edmonton-based Hotel de Health announced it wanted to lease a closed hospital in the Red Deer area to offer private hospital care, Clay Adams, communications director for Alberta's East Central Health Authority, said it could become a source of badly needed revenues. "To have a health care centre sitting empty is unproductive," Adams said. "If we can find an alternative use we should."

Alberta was also the home of the Health Resources Group, the 37-bed, for-profit, Calgary hospital described in chapter 9. In May 1997, federal Health Minister David Dingwall warned Alberta Premier Ralph Klein that if Klein didn't stop the opening of the for-profit hospital, he would. Instead the Canadian Medical Discovery Fund, a joint project of the federal government's Medical Research Council and health corporation MDS, gave HRG $2 million in start up capital. HRG promised to sell private medical services to the Workers' Compensation Board, private corporations, Americans, native groups, and others.[22]

The pattern established in the United States, a pattern that is leading to an integration of nonprofit and for-profit medicine, has moved north of the border. Although public-private partnerships between nonprofit and for-profit Canadian hospitals have occurred on a limited scale, as hospitals continue to be battered by funding shortfalls and cutbacks they are actively looking for new revenue.

In 1994 St. Joseph's Hospital in London, Ontario, established what it called a "unique partnership" with Dynacare, an integrated health-services company with extensive holdings in the U.S., to open the Pall Mall Rehabilitation Clinic. Profits from the joint venture were to be shared between the hospital and the company, supplementing St. Joseph's reduced provincial funding. The hospital said the new rehab centre would differentiate itself from other providers by offering "compassionate treatment ... while recognizing and meeting the requirements of its financial sponsors."

St. Joseph's was one of the first in Canada to get involved in for-profit health care, but it wouldn't be the last. As the government of Mike Harris moved aggressively down the road pioneered by Alberta with hospital closures around the province and continued funding cutbacks, it forced administrators, favourably disposed towards the corporate sector to begin with, to search for alternative sources of revenue in for-profit health-care ventures.

THIRTEEN

MDS Inc., Canada's Home-Grown Behemoth

MDS Inc., is Canada's largest and most aggressive health- and life-sciences corporation and one of the country's most interesting companies. Founded in Toronto in 1969 as Medical Data Sciences, Ltd., by five former employees of IBM's medical services division, the company originally intended to provide health screening services to large Ontario employers. Since then it has played an influential role in supporting – in fact, in creating – a private health market in Canada for its products and services, and in capturing a sizable portion of the money allocated by the public for health services.

MDS's modest beginnings can be traced to the west end of Toronto, where the company purchased four labs known as Toronto Medical Laboratories Ltd. to support its health screening business. In less than fifteen years, MDS had secured a footing in strategic sectors of the North American health-care market and was a leading global merchant of services, medical equipment, and sophisticated analytical instrumentation. Today seven divisions carry the company's logo from coast to coast and around the world: MDS Laboratory Services, MDS Ingram and Bell, MDS Nordion, MDS Communicare, MDS SCIEX, MDS Pharmaceutical Services, and MDS Capital Corp. MDS Capital manages five venture capital arms: MDS Health Ventures Inc., the Health Care and Biotechnology Venture Fund, the Neurosciences Partners Limited Partnership, the B.C. Life Sciences Fund, and the Canadian Medical Discoveries Fund. Together these funds command over $400 million in both public and private development money, providing start-up capital to a range of companies, many of them emerging as part of the MDS empire. More than forty new health companies have benefitted from $94 million in MDS Capital start-up funding, and this funding has purchased direct equity shares for MDS in many of the new entities.

With 45 percent of its $819 million in revenues earned outside of the country in 1996, MDS is as eager to go out into the global health market as it is to establish and nurture a health-care marketplace in Canada. In this endeavour, as in all others MDS Inc. has involved itself in, the profit potential has been carefully assessed, strategies developed, and the necessary steps taken to expand its reach and the company's earnings. Canadian sensitivity to health-care profits has required MDS to go to great lengths to justify the money it siphons out of the health system and into the pockets of shareholders. One oft-repeated argument is that investors must earn a profit to offset the risk they take with their money.[1]

The company's market is divided among three sectors: health-care providers, including hospitals and private insurers, provide 55 percent of revenues; manufacturers, such as pharmaceutical and biotechnology companies, contribute 39 percent to revenues; and consumers, who use rehabilitative and home health-care products supplied by MDS, contribute 6 percent annually to its gross income.

There have been very few serious setbacks in MDS's short history, reflecting a cautious management style coupled with a sophisticated analysis of the potential for private-sector expansion in Canada's huge health-care market. These characteristics have been complemented by strategic alliances with like-minded corporate players and an aggressive pursuit of key relationships with governments at both the federal and provincial levels. MDS and its many partners, both in the corporate and nonprofit sectors, have focussed their combined energies on "growing" the private health market in Canada. Physicians played a key role in the company's earlier years, providing its laboratories, in particular, with medical expertise in diagnostic procedures. This association increased MDS's credibility and, just as importantly, the number of patients referred to its labs for blood testing. Today, however, doctors have less significance in the overall strategies than other, more important links that have developed during the 1990s.

MDS's partnering has increasingly occurred with Canadian, U.S., Asian and European corporations such as Dupont Merck, the Pfizer Corporation, Bristol Meyer-Squibb, BCE Inc., Manulife, Dynacare, Columbia/HCA, Liberty, the Allegiance Corporation, HealthStreams, the Royal Bank of Canada, and British Aerospace. It has diligently pursued both formal and informal joint ventures with hospitals in Canada and the United States and is actively involved in federal, provincial, and regional government discussions about issues ranging from utilization protocols, outsourcing, information systems technology, and spending to export strategies and trade rules. In addition, the company has cultivated productive relationships with politicians and bureaucrats of every political persuasion, who, according to MDS president John Rogers, "have changed their attitude to private health care companies" in the era of fiscal restraint.[2]

From the beginning

It was anybody's guess in the late 1960s whether the group of five entrepreneurs who founded MDS could survive in Canada, with its traditional public antipathy towards companies that profited from the ills and ailments of vulnerable patients. The private sector always has been present in Canada's health-care delivery and insurance systems, although the insurance industry's reach was curtailed sharply with the introduction of medicare. The development, manufacture, and distribution of drugs, sophisticated technology, and medical and surgical supplies and equipment were colonized permanently by private companies that relied on generous infusions of public money and supplier contracts from governments and health-care institutions. But the private-lab sector, MDS's original target, was relatively fragmented in Ontario where, as in other provinces, publicly insured outpatient diagnostic testing occurred mainly in hospitals. When it became clear the market opportunities for employee health screening were minimal, MDS refocussed its energy on the lab business.

In 1973, when it burst onto the Toronto Stock Exchange as a publicly traded company named MDS Health Group Ltd., it was forging a path to what company officials would later describe as a "diversified technology-based health care organization." The firm would play a major role in developing in Canada what did not exist when it started out: a large, for-profit, corporate-driven market for its array of products and services. It was an environment in which MDS would come to exemplify the negative relationship between public funding cutbacks and a deteriorating public policy framework on the one hand, and the shift in delivery of services from a cost-controlled nonprofit environment to a profit-focussed – and therefore more costly and competitive – health-care marketplace on the other.[3]

MDS's greatest asset in the early years of its history was its ability to tap the pool of public health dollars for outpatient diagnostic services funded by Ontario's health-insurance plan. Prior to 1967, when Ontario agreed to participate in the national health program, private laboratories were individually owned, usually by a physician, and testing was paid for by private insurers or patients. When MDS was founded in 1969, private labs had been brought into the public health-care system and were funded on a fee-for-service, or per test, basis by the medical plan. This payment method was not extended to hospitals, which included outpatient lab services in their global budgets, funded by ministries of health. This public-private split in payment for diagnostic testing was eventually adopted by most provinces that allowed private labs to operate. It established a division between inpatient and outpatient services and reinforced it with two separate payment schemes: one, fee-for-service, for private labs; the other, annual funding, for hospitals.

The public-private split was reinforced, as well, by the development of sophisticated technology for the delivery of lab services. Technology transformed what once were manually intensive, routine lab procedures into rapid, automated specimen analyses. Technological change greatly assisted community-based clinics' routine testing of patients, but this left hospitals with the more complicated, labour-intensive, and expensive analytical procedures that private laboratories often were not equipped or qualified to handle. In addition, patients admitted to hospital often were in a more acute stage of illness than outpatients, whose testing was done by the growing number of private facilities. A final twist was that the payment method – fee-for-service for routine, less expensive testing – gave private labs access to a steady source of revenue from the public purse, which offered incentives to test liberally. This situation, which set up a false division between the respective roles of public and private labs, put diagnostic testing on the leading edge in the transfer of outpatient services from increasingly cash-strapped hospitals to large, profit-focussed corporations.[4]

In 1972, when MDS was well into its plan to bring many of Ontario's independent, physician-owned labs into its fold, the company had established the modus operandi that would become its hallmark. Its aggressive expansion in Ontario's lab sector was accomplished by acquisitions, investments, amalgamations, partnerships, and share transfers to or between the growing number of subsidiaries. In 1978 MDS Health Group and ten of its wholly-owned subsidiaries amalgamated, and the company continued its strategy of buying up smaller companies throughout Ontario. Profits during this time were compounding by an estimated 18 to 20 percent per year, and 80 percent of revenues were derived from public fee-for-service payments for diagnostic services. As MDS's revenues in the lab sector increased, the amount of money received by hospitals for the same services declined.[5]

The growth experienced by MDS during the 1980s and 1990s was remarkable, enabling the company to accelerate its movement into other parts of the health sector. Much of this growth was made possible not by the creation of "new" markets, but rather by the redirection of patients from the hospital sector to MDS and other private labs. As private labs expanded their presence in Ontario and other provinces, lab fees increased and usage rates skyrocketed. In every province with significant private-sector participation, costs for diagnostic testing soared, while the percentage of outpatient tests performed in the hospital sector declined.

The use of lab services increased from an average 10.96 tests per person in 1979/80 to 19.01 in 1990/91 in Ontario. But per capita costs for those services during the same period increased by more than 300 percent, from $33.29 to $100.19, the highest rate in the country, consuming 6.6 percent of total health expenditures. There were 173 private labs in the province in 1991, receiving $428.1 million in payments from the Ontario Health Insurance Plan, compared with receipts of $112.3 million ten years earlier and $63.2 million in 1976-77. Like Ontario, Alberta, Saskatchewan, British Columbia, and Manitoba all had seen a rapid expansion of private-sector activity, paralleled by substantial increases in costs and utilization of lab services. Not coincidentally, these provinces had higher per capita costs than Québec, Nova Scotia, New Brunswick, Newfoundland, and Prince Edward Island, where private labs were not permitted to duplicate the insured services offered by nonprofit hospitals.[6]

As provincial governments began feeling the impact of reduced federal funds for health in the early 1990s, they turned their attention to reducing the cost and use of publicly funded health-care services, including diagnostic testing. Not a single government in the country, not even NDP administrations with their party's traditional commitment to public delivery of health services, attempted to reduce the amount of publicly funded testing done in MDS and other private labs. The increased cost/use problems were common in every province, "and none of them knows what to do about it," commented Dr. Dennis Pstuka, former Ontario assistant deputy minister of health, in 1991. "The attempts to regulate the private lab industry have all been resounding failures." Though the rate of increase in the fees paid by OHIP to private labs, described variously as "dramatic" and "alarming," had never been examined by the province, the situation was becoming critical by the early 1990s. While admitting they did not know the reasons for rising private-sector lab billings to OHIP, health ministry officials agreed that "We have to look at exactly what is causing this."[7]

The government consulted the private sector in its search for answers. John Rogers, a top executive at MDS and chair of the Ontario Association of Medical Laboratories (which the company had helped organize), said, "We think the growth in laboratory expenditures is explainable": 7 percent of doctors queried in an MDS survey said they ordered tests because they feared malpractice suits by patients; 38 percent of patients requested tests they had heard about, leading physicians to order inappropriately; testing among twenty- to fifty-year-olds, 75 percent of whom were women "in their child-bearing, menopausal or post-menopausal years" (in other words, all women) had seen the most rapid rate of increase; and up to 80 percent more tests were ordered for males per patient visit. No mention was made by Rogers as to whether MDS had played a role in increased use, or whether its rising profit margins, most of which were derived from the lab revenues collected from OHIP, might be to blame.[8]

There was, in addition, a direct correlation between higher lab costs and physicians' simultaneous involvement in both the public and private sectors. After diagnostic laboratories in Alberta were reorganized into a regional structures, for example, it was found that in two regions where pathologists did not maintain investments in, or close ties with, the private-laboratory sector, the volume of testing dropped by 25 percent after the doctors initiated a use-management program. In British Columbia, the only province where both hospital and private-sector outpatient testing was funded on a fee-for-service basis, it was found that some physicians, "in addition to owning and operating private diagnostic facilities, also have considerable influence, through their positions on the staffs of hospitals in their own community, over the activities of the hospital facilities with which they compete" for public funds. These physicians could decide where to refer patients for blood testing and acted as mediators in the complex relationships that existed between public and private facilities and among private labs. Such dual roles for doctors invested in the lab sector raised a host of conflict of interest concerns.[9]

The early relationship between MDS and physicians was a strategic one for the company. In the early 1970s it established a Medical Advisory Board within its Lab Services Division. By the mid-1990s this board was composed of up to 100 physicians – both those employed by the company as well as those working in private practice – to oversee all clinical aspects of the operation. In this way, MDS assured investors, it was "meeting the needs of the health care system, as well as developing a network of medical intelligence" giving the company "an insight into emerging health care trends and technologies." The company also appointed a locally based pathologist to serve as medical director in each of its laboratories, boasting that "in most cases these pathologists also serve as medical directors of hospital laboratories in their communities." This professional partnership, MDS officials said, was a "key to [its] success," opening doors "between the company and government, between the company and the medical profession, between the company and institutions in the health care field, including hospitals and university medical establishments." The strategy helped boost MDS to become the largest lab operator in Ontario and, soon after, in the country.[10]

The professional partnership with physicians was, indeed, instrumental to MDS's success as a laboratory services provider, beginning in Ontario and spreading west to Saskatchewan, Alberta and British Columbia during the 1980s and 1990s. It was useful to have medical men on the team who understood the discipline and who could relate to the physicians whose laboratories were targeted in MDS's expansion strategies in the fragmented Canadian market. The appointment of Dr. John Nixon as the first MDS Laboratories medical director in 1972 provided the company with a vigilant advocate in the medical community and helped solidify the relationship with physicians, many of whom would be referring patients to the private lab for testing. These efforts were supported by the publication of company materials that were distributed to doctors. These dealt with a broad array of issues, including questions of appropriate testing, diagnosis, and care.[11]

Lab services in the 1990s

Regionalization and provincial cutbacks to the hospital sector were opening up opportunities for MDS across the country during the 1990s. Revenues jumped to $640 million in 1993, a 44 percent increase over the previous year. But in the same year, Ontario announced a 20 percent reduction in laboratory fees over the next four years. Although the fee reductions were minuscule in comparison to the nearly 300 percent increase in private-sector lab revenues from 1981 to

1991, the company could see the writing on the wall. It negotiated multiyear pricing agreements with Ontario, B.C., Alberta, and Saskatchewan to help stabilize revenue expectations from the sector. At the same time it decided it had to diversify, reorganize, and wean itself from dependence on outpatient lab revenues if it was to stay in the game. "We have anticipated, and continue to anticipate, that funding for health care will be under severe pressures," said Ron Yamada, vice president and one of the founders of MDS.

The company underwent a $26-million restructuring in its core lab and medical supply businesses, digging into profits. For the first three months of 1994, MDS painted a picture of distress while it continued centralizing operations and accelerating development of its automated lab equipment. In January the company predicted it would cut 200 jobs across the country, adding to 200 lab positions already eliminated. But five top MDS officers "shared the pain" being experienced by shareholders, if not employees. Chairman Wilf Lewitt's income was cut from $289,750 to $283,625, and although he received stock options worth $432,000, his bonus fell from $99,750 to $72,675. MDS President John Rogers, along with four senior vice presidents, saw their incomes reduced to $235,758 each, down from almost $250,000, a blow that was ameliorated somewhat by stock options worth $216,000 each.[12] But, "Innovation," proclaimed a headline in the Toronto *Star*, was "the daughter of necessity" at MDS. By April the worst was over. Soaring health costs, Lewitt told shareholders at the company's annual meeting, were creating opportunities, and cuts in government spending had moved the company to develop other aspects of the business.

The company wasn't about to abandon its laboratory division, though. Instead MDS began developing an automated robotics system to handle 70 percent of specimens, which would no longer need to be touched by a single human hand. The system became operational in late 1994.[13] The launch of this new $10 million subsidiary, AutoLab, in the Laboratory Services Division positioned MDS to move beyond its base as a mere blood-testing company and into the more lucrative product supplier and lab management end of the business. MDS claimed that the automated system would substantially reduce its largest cost component – labour – when it was installed in its Etobicoke head office at the end of the year. Having weathered the storm, and with more than $100 million in cash, MDS was once again "looking for acquisitions in the health care field."[14]

In fact, the automated lab system was the company's ticket into, not out of, Canada's tightened public purse. Developed by MDS laboratory employees, the system used equipment manufactured by the AutoMed Corporation, another MDS subsidiary based in Richmond, B.C., and a specimen transportation system provided by Automated Tooling Systems, Inc. (ATS), of Cambridge, Ontario. (Ironically, ATS, whose main customers were automobile companies, credited its robotics technology with a decision to cancel outsourcing contracts that cost more than in-house production.) AutoLab's robotic, computerized lab testing technology had its first trial run at the MDS lab in Etobicoke, where approximately half the laboratory technologists were laid off, victims of a 300 percent increase in productivity – an increase of questionable necessity in a market considered to be operating in overdrive.[15]

When MDS installed the automated lab system at the world-renowned Mayo Clinic in 1993 it was a "sales breakthrough in the important U.S. market," and one that led the company to initiate a careful strategy to sell the idea in a global market estimated to be worth $500 million. MDS said the equipment, which could double or triple productivity in most labs, "can substantially reduce costs to the health care system," while offering substantial revenues to the company. The opening of a new Toronto medical laboratory in a 50-50 joint venture with The Toronto Hospital fit nicely with the company's global strategy and was announced with great fanfare despite the sad news that many TTH lab employees would lose their jobs.[16]

By 1994, the company was operating 400 of its own labs, as well as a growing number located in hospitals. During the 1990s it also entered lucrative partnerships with universities, hospitals, governments, and several multinational corporations, providing clinical trial drug tests, diagnostic services, environmental testing, medical product distribution, and an array of paramedical and home-care services. The company had opened its doors in every region of the country, with the exception of the Atlantic provinces, and had another seven locations in the United States. In addition, MDS could be found in Belgium,

Northern Ireland, the United Kingdom, Germany, Switzerland, the United Arab Republic, Hong Kong, Japan, Taiwan, and China.[17]

Its dependence on income from the lab sector was quickly decreasing, but lab reimbursement fees from public coffers still contributed one third of the company's overall revenue and 40 percent of its profits. The continuing squeeze by governments on outpatient testing led MDS to begin an aggressive and controversial pursuit of inpatient diagnostic services, aimed at both hospitals and regional health boards in several provinces. "If we are going to meet the challenge of cost containment and quality of care," said Alan Torrie, president of MDS Laboratories and former CEO of Joseph Brant Hospital in Burlington, Ontario, "we have to build bridges between the public and private sectors in a constructive way."

In 1996 MDS negotiated an agreement with the Calgary Regional Health Authority that helped the company build a bridge into a deeper pool of public funds. The company was contracted by the regional health authority to integrate and manage all hospital and private-sector lab services in the region. While noting the tough times government cost cutting had imposed on the company (but which had not dampened its profits), MDS said its Laboratory Services Division had been able to adapt. "An example of successful adjustment is the Alberta experience," the company's 1997 annual report stated. "MDS had its own laboratory operation in Calgary with revenues of $26 million a year ... Now, MDS has become the managing partner of a much larger joint venture with revenues of $70 million a year."[18]

Although some were skeptical about the company's "constructive partnership" theories, there was a cheering section in the investment community. The nonprofit sector, said Marian Pitters, a Toronto management consultant, didn't have a corner on goodness "just because they don't make a profit." Quality and efficiency counted too, a fact that was finally being recognized, she said, by hospital administrators. "On the one side there's social entrepreneurialism where people in the private sector want to make a contribution to what's happening in the community," she said. "On the other side there's an entrepreneurial socialism afoot in the not-for-profit sector as [administrators] understand that in order to survive the financial crunch they must be creative and innovative in generating revenue and can't look at funds coming from the government as something they're entitled to." Never mind that a growing number of "social entrepreneurs" were dipping their hands in the public till and were now competing with nonprofit health-care providers for limited funds.[19]

Fiscal belt-tightening in the health-care sector, MDS had informed its employees in 1993, was forcing the company to do more with less. "We may not have had much say in the creation of the deficit problem," it said, ignoring its own role in escalating lab costs, "but we are compelled to carry part of the burden." Ontario's move to cut $246 million from the health-care system had triggered an angry response from public-sector workers, who rejected the government's call for an agreement to cut their wages. Instead the workers' unions demanded that work done in private labs be shifted to the hospital sector for a potential saving of $200 million. This claim was supported by a 1991 Ministry of Health study that concluded private-sector labs were 34 percent more costly than their hospital counterparts.

Despite the insistence in the business press that governments cut spending on public services and use the savings to pay down the deficit, the *Financial Post* decried the unions' cost-saving proposal and their "blind commitment to enforce a publicly funded, nonprofit medical laboratory system." Private labs, according to an editorial in the paper, "have an enviable record of innovation" and "are a dynamic segment of the health-care system, one of which the Ontario government should be proud." It was a curious display of the contradictions in the ideology of conservative leaders, two of whose main planks – lower health-care spending and increased for-profit, private involvement in the sector – appeared to cancel one another out.[20]

The protestations in the business press reflected the views of MDS, which said the private sector "has already suffered through the recession in ways that the public sector and its employees have not." Yet despite its suffering, "our industry has been specifically targeted by public sector employee spokesmen as one that should be further attacked by government." The company clearly was worried, charging that public-sector unions had "urged that testing ... be taken out of the private sector and turned over to hospitals or other public sector agencies." If that happened, MDS warned, it would damage its own interests as well as those of other companies in the lab business. "Ontario is only one jurisdiction," the company warned, but other provinces "either have taken or may in the future take approaches similar to those being urged on Ontario. So we have reason to be concerned."[21]

The similar approaches MDS worried about were being examined in British Columbia two years later. MDS had moved across the Rocky Mountains and into the province in April 1987 with a 50 percent acquisition of Metro-McNair Clinical Laboratories, a move that led to a significant presence in Canada's three westernmost provinces. Metro-McNair itself was the result of a merger between Metropolitan Clinical Laboratories and McNair Laboratories in 1961. Metropolitan was founded by John Nixon and two partners to conduct thyroid tests not offered by B.C. hospitals. A year after the lab opened its doors, Dr. Don Rix joined the company as a partner and in 1969 became a shareholder in McNair Laboratories when its owner sold the business. During the years that followed, Metro-McNair competed fiercely with hospital laboratories for patient referrals from the province's physicians, developing strong loyalties among many members of the B.C. Medical Association, which eventually came to negotiate on behalf of private labs for access to funds from the Medical Services Commission. Nixon, who by this time was medical director at MDS, and Rix, now head of the merged Vancouver labs, had maintained a close friendship through the years, which was helpful when discussions for a partnership between Metro-McNair and MDS first arose.[22]

MDS's stake in Metro-McNair increased to 75 percent in 1992, after a buying spree lasting several years had stretched the Vancouver lab's reach into Edmonton, Calgary, Regina, and Winnipeg. At the time there were three large private companies in B.C. that owned a majority of the 134 private laboratories and 78 specimen-collection centres around the province: Metro-McNair, B.C. Biomedical, and Island Medical Laboratories. In 1995 MDS bought Island Medical, bringing the bulk of Vancouver Island diagnostic services under its corporate umbrella. Unlike the system in most other provinces, both hospitals and private labs were paid on a fee-for-service basis for outpatient lab work billed to the medical plan. In total, private labs billed the plan almost $176 million, while hospitals were responsible for just over $59 million in outpatient laboratory billings.

The large expenditures for diagnostic services, most of which went to MDS, and the "overcapacity" identified in the sector, led Elizabeth Cull, the minister of health at the time, to appoint a review commission headed by Dr. Miles Kilshaw to study the situation and report back with recommendations. Kilshaw's well-researched report, issued in March 1994, contained several recommendations that were guaranteed to arouse the ire of the BCMA and the private-lab sector. In a detailed discussion of the province's diagnostic laboratories (blood and urine), medical imaging (X-ray, CT scans, MRI), electrodiagnostics (for example, electrocardiograms), and pulmonary function testing (lungs), the report outlined the problems that had led to a half-billion-dollar annual outlay for services. Kilshaw cited problems including the lack of accountability in the private sector and the fee-for-service remuneration of physicians and both public and private laboratories. Conflict of interest, the report said, was common where physicians who played critical roles in hospital pathology departments maintained ownership or shares in companies that benefitted from a high volume of testing. "In addition," the Kilshaw report noted, "the owners and operators of some of these private facilities are prominent in the hierarchy and committee structure of the BCMA, which ... sets the fees charged" for diagnostic services. The BCMA negotiated the fee schedule on behalf of hospitals and private laboratories, the report stated, rather than acting for the pathologists employed in the facilities. Furthermore, physicians who were involved in the accreditation or monitoring of laboratories were "placed in the position of reviewing the activities of facilities with which they may be competing," leading to potential conflicts of interest.[23]

The report also criticized the absence of regulatory controls over the opening of new private labs – whether they were needed in the community or not – as well as "large gaps in the overseeing of diagnostic facilities." Rules and regulations "appear to emphasize maximum access, rather than optimal utilization or need," while changes in "facilities, equipment, ownership, and service delivery" had occurred without the knowledge of the Medical Services Commission (MSC), which was responsible for licensing and payment to laboratories. The MSC did not collect information "as to where a specimen or test is provided," and regulations did not exist "concerning the expansion of diagnostic services already provided." There were no "appropriate penalties for violation of policies or billing guidelines," while the MSC was unable to prevent inappropriate billings by "non-approved physicians under the name of one who is approved."[24]

The report contained dozens of recommendations. Three in particular sent the private labs into a panic. The first urged the government to implement a strategy to bring diagnostic services back into the hospital sector where public control could exert a positive impact on costs. The second recommendation called for the establishment of an agency to oversee the allocation of funds and licensing for diagnostic services, removing that responsibility from the BCMA-dominated Medical Services Commission. A third recommendation called for conflict-of-interest guidelines to ensure that physicians did not profit from their patient referrals to labs in which they owned shares. In 1995, shortly after the report was released, Paul Ramsey, who had inherited the health portfolio from Cull, rejected these three recommendations out of hand. Soon after, the entire report was consigned to a back shelf amidst rumours that "what happened to Kilshaw was MDS."

When the Kilshaw report was released, MDS was developing its government relations in B.C. Its strategy, applied effectively in Saskatchewan and Alberta Fas well, involved a persistent and aggressive courting of elected and nonelected government officials. After the B.C. government buried Kilshaw's report in 1995, it entered into a public-private partnership with MDS, establishing a $20 million venture capital fund. The B.C. Life Sciences Fund received half of its original capital from the province's Treasury Board, headed by the new finance minister, Elizabeth Cull. Another $5 million was thrown in by the Royal Bank, with the remainder contributed by MDS, which would manage the fund's investment portfolio. MDS also was awarded a contract to manage six technology-based companies included in another government-backed fund called Discovery Enterprises. Glen Clark, the province's future premier, hoped the new initiative would help "diversify [B.C.'s] economy away from the traditional area of resource extraction" and develop "the value-added jobs of the future." A year later, Cull was defeated in a provincial election and was soon working as a consultant for the company.[25]

Public funds in the corporate sector

It was in public-private partnerships that MDS saw its future. "Sharing the burden," (but not the profits) was the MDS theme of the 1980s and 1990s. In 1987 MDS had challenged critics who asked, "Why should private companies be allowed to make a profit out of the illness of people?" The company called this a "loaded question" (as opposed to a good one), which reflected a widespread attitude that MDS was prepared to tackle.

There were problems in trying to assess "the financial pros and cons" between private- and public-sector operations, the company asserted, including different accounting systems that "sometimes led to misleading comparisons." It claimed the private sector had made investments in health and social services that governments were reluctant to make without increasing taxes substantially. The fundamental question facing society was "not about the ownership of health care service systems, or about the earning of reasonable profits by investors," but rather was "about the quality and availability of the services and their real costs." The privatization trend around the globe, said MDS, "acknowledges the legitimacy of profit as a reward for risk, for effort and for efficient, effective provision of goods and services."[26]

Not surprisingly, MDS's first hospital joint venture occurred in the United States, where profit in health care was not a dirty word. The partnership with two nonprofit facilities in New York's Hudson River Valley region provided MDS with experience it could later apply in its home territory. Hospital Shared Services (HSS) was founded in 1980 as a core lab integrating the inpatient and outpatient testing services of four hospitals in the area. By pooling their resources, these hospitals hoped to realize substantial savings. Despite five years of planning among the four facilities, the joint venture had difficulty establishing itself. One hospital dropped out soon after the launch, while another declared bankruptcy a few years later, adding to the financial strains being felt at the time. The two remaining partners, Vassar Brothers and Northern Duchess, remained committed to the project. But the lab continued to lurch from one problem to another, including an inexperienced management team that was unable to effectively market the lab's services and a lack of "outreach services" – including computer links to physician offices and collection sites, the lifeblood, so to speak, of the lab business.

In 1986 MDS approached HSS about a joint venture, and HSS jumped, giving the Canadian company a management contract to operate the lab. A year later, the board of directors decided to invite proposals from some of the largest commercial labs in the U.S., as well as MDS, to either manage HSS or enter a joint venture agreement. "But it was a Canadian lab, MDS, which ended up as our chosen partner," said Ron Mullahey, president of Vassar Brothers Hospital.

In 1995, MDS Vice President Robert Brecken recalled why his company was so interested in the Hudson Valley. "Our original intent was threefold," he said. "First, we see the United States ... as a leading indicator of some of the changes to health care in Canada, particularly in laboratory and hospital operations. Thus, working within the United States provides us with experience and knowledge on new developments that we can carry into Canada." The company also wanted to keep its toe in U.S. waters, he said, because it "keeps us current and up-to-date should we wish to re-enter the U.S. market under a new operating model in the future." The third reason was the opportunities inherent in HSS, "given the geography and catchment area," for revenue growth and profits. "We think of this as a business that can really grow and return a reasonable profit to the shareholders over the long term," Brecken said.

In 1988 MDS closed its lab in nearby Kingston, New York, and bought a 50 percent share of HSS, triggering both a change of name and status at the same time. Vassar Brothers Hospital now held 32 percent of the shares, while Northern Duchess held 18 percent, making MDS the largest single shareholder in the joint venture. Hudson Shared Services was reborn as MDS-Hudson Valley Laboratories, Inc.

(MDS-HVL), a for-profit entity. "You really cannot run a tax-exempt [nonprofit] company in a for-profit environment," said Mullahey, a fair warning for those in Canada who supported an expansion of private-sector involvement in health-care delivery as a way to ease the burden on the country's single-payer, nonprofit system.

When MDS-HVL recorded its first profits in 1994, tensions arose among the company's directors. "The board of directors has a difficult time with this conflict about profit," said Glen Fine, newly appointed general manager of MDS-HVL. Eventually MDS would want to see a return on its investment "in the form of regular profit distributions," but the hospitals' interests lay in using the profits to reduce lab costs. "This is a real challenge," Brecken said. Unlike MDS, the hospitals were involved in the lab to minimize their costs, but "we want to have a profit that can be shared among the shareholders and re-invested in the business." Despite these differing perspectives, Brecken said, "balance among these different priorities is what this partnership is all about," adding that "as a financial investor, we have reason to anticipate a healthy financial return in the future."[27]

By 1992 the company was reshaping its participation in the U.S. market, having sold its substantial network of clinical laboratories in New York state, Pennsylvania, and New Jersey for more than U.S.$50 million to Corning Lab Services in 1991. Corning, which pleaded guilty in late 1996 to charges it had defrauded Medicare of tens of millions of dollars, planned to merge MDS's operation into its subsidiary, MetPath, Inc., "a company with an outstanding reputation in the ... industry," according to MDS President John Rogers. But MDS retained its investment in the Hudson Valley lab, which by 1996 boasted three hospital partners, eight licensed laboratories, twenty patient service centres, twenty-four long-term care facilities under full-service contracts, 300 employees, and anticipated annual revenues of between US$20 million and $25 million. MDS-HVL became the dominant lab provider in the area by 1994, generating "an acceptable level of profit and ROI." Even more importantly, it had "significant value as a salable asset" when the opportunity presented itself.[28]

However, in mid-1997, Local 1199 of the National Health and Human Services Employees Union began raising question about the ties between nonprofit Vassar Brothers and for-profit MDS, charging that the hospital, with "an exclusive contract to provide services to its patients with a company that it has part ownership in," was involved in a conflict of interest and a possible violation of Medicare and Medicaid regulations. The arrangement, said the union, "creates an incentive for the hospital to order unnecessary blood work – ultimately raising health care costs in this area." It added that the compensation and financial incentives paid to Vassar Brothers' president, Ron Mullahey, "remain unclear at this time." The union, a leader in the fight for nonprofit health care in the U.S., continues to query the relationship between the hospital and MDS.[29]

It was only a matter of time before MDS carried into Canada the experience it had gained working in the United States. The company had entered into a number of agreements in Ontario's hospital sector, the first as early as 1986 with Toronto General Hospital shortly before its merger with Western to form The Toronto Hospital (TTH). The partnership established Health and Research Services, Inc., to fund the development and commercialization of orthopedic products and diagnostic testing procedures. It was the beginning of a lucrative and long-term relationship with Canada's largest teaching and research hospital, one that would help "lever" other opportunities with other similar facilities.

The Toronto Hospital, like almost all hospitals in Canada, is independently owned but operates with public funds on a nonprofit basis, providing insured services in accordance with provincial legislation. Linked to the University of Toronto, TTH manages 1200 beds and an annual budget of more than $500 million, with over 37,000 patient admissions a year. In 1993, with public-sector health expenditures declining by 0.3 percent, TTH and other hospitals turned to the private sector, where health spending had increased by 7.2 percent in the same year, for ideas about how to save – and raise – money.[30]

Like many hospital administrators, those at TTH were predisposed towards the "free market" when they decided in 1993 that "the support services functions of the hospital could be carried out at less cost" by private companies. Hospitals, wrote three top TTH executives in a review of the facility's experience with public-private partnerships, "simply cannot compete with the economies of scale enjoyed by business," particularly those with worldwide operations and a low-paid workforce.

The decision to do business with the private sector was buttressed with elaborate explanations about the "certain discrete products or services" that formed the core mission of The Toronto Hospital. TTH was constructing a "new lexicon" that included words like outsourcing which, it said, occurred when a "company," such as a hospital, "determines that it cannot, or should not, be engaged in a certain business ... Hence, the notion of 'core competencies' − the identification of the essential or core businesses of the company." Administrators went to great and complicated lengths to explain why they were outsourcing services that the hospital had successfully managed since its inception: "The creation of these end products," they wrote, "requires the application of many intermediate products or services which may represent the core competencies of other companies who are desirous of selling these products or services (as an end product) to another company (that will use them as an intermediate product) to produce an end product."[31]

What were these "end products" produced in the hospital sector? According to Michael Young, chief financial officer at Toronto's Sunnybrook Hospital, it was a well patient, one that could be "built" more efficiently if administrators understood their product costs. "There are some aspects of health care that can be compared with a manufacturing organization," said Young. "The process is patient care; the output is well patients."[32]

An assessment of "product costs" by TTH drew it to the self-evident fact that hospitals are labour-intensive organizations and that most of the savings that would accrue to TTH from its relationships with the corporate sector "will be derived from this category." While seniority provisions in collective agreements made the layoff of hospital workers disruptive, TTH said dismissively, "Seniority, per se, is increasingly of marginal importance." It looked forward to labour code changes announced by Ontario's new Conservative government − changes that would "provide for greater labour management flexibility" and allow the hospital to outsource and lay off, unhindered by contract obligations to its 6000 employees.[33]

The savings realized by TTH came almost entirely from the pockets of employees, both those whose jobs were outsourced by the hospital and those working in the private sector at substantially lower wages who took over the outsourced functions. The elusive "economies of scale" so envied by public administrators at TTH apparently could not be achieved in an environment governed by collective agreements, but there was some contradiction apparent in the hospital's discomfort with contracts negotiated with its employees and its attitude to those it concluded with the private sector. The "best contract [with private companies]," the executives said, was "one which follows careful due diligence." However, because hospitals must recognize "the legitimate right of a partner to earn a healthy rate of return on their investment," the best contract should not be used "as a fulcrum to force either partner to live up to the other's expectations." If there was a "trade-off between capturing operating costs and quality or service levels," the administrators cautioned, hospitals must be prepared "to support that trade-off."[34]

While outsourcing was an attractive, if cumbersome, method of reducing costs, of growing interest to TTH was the opportunity to generate alternative sources of revenue to offset funding reductions by the provincial government. This shift – from saving money to generating revenues – was a significant one that threatened the principle of nonprofit delivery of medically necessary services in Canada's hospital sector. The shift was taking place among a number of hospitals throughout the province, almost entirely without public oversight or even public awareness. As mentioned in chapter 12, for example, St. Joseph's Hospital in London, Ontario, had pioneered a joint venture with Dynacare, a multinational health-services company and rival of MDS, to set up the Pall Mall Rehabilitation Clinic in February 1994. The new facility, according to St. Joseph's, would "differentiate itself from other providers by offering compassionate treatment tailored to individual needs while recognizing and meeting the requirements of financial sponsors" – a kinder, gentler way of saying the clinic would operate as a for-profit enterprise. A year later, after Dynacare began negotiations to take over testing at Sunnybrook hospital, MDS and TTH announced they would be setting up the "Lab of the Future," using MDS's automated robotics technology. MDS Chairman Wilf Lewitt said he hoped the joint venture would use the company's expertise at cutting the jobs of laboratory staff and retraining those who remained, skills it had learned during a year of restructuring and technological change at its own business. "We have been through the anguish of downsizing, so we can help in the complete implementation of the system in other businesses," said Lewitt.[35]

The transition from outsourcing to partnership arrangements was a predictable one, and though it "meant that the Hospital would have to shoulder ... higher levels of risk" than its corporate partners, it was "generally felt that traditional outsourcing arrangements, while generally 'safe', would only yield traditional returns." TTH was looking for "nontraditional returns." It needed revenue, a difficult pursuit for nonprofit health-care institutions, but one that was winning converts as provincial funding dried up and as administrators became the subjects of an aggressive sales pitch from the corporate sector. If TTH failed to achieve that goal, hospital executives warned, it "would almost surely mean the dramatic downsizing or elimination of some of the Hospital's clinical offerings."

With this in mind, TTH joined a growing number of hospitals across the country that were interested in creating new for-profit joint ventures with private corporations. Among the hospital's new partners were the Bitove Corporation, providing "kitchenless" food services; Johnson Controls, supplying housekeeping, grounds and waste management, security, transportation, and support services; and Searle Canada, subsidiary of U.S. chemical and drug company, Monsanto. "Partnerships with corporate sponsors such as Searle Canada are essential to help us compete," said Dr. Alan Hudson, head of TTH. If there were those who wondered what nonprofit hospitals were competing for, the answer was money, an increasing portion of which was derived from profits generated in the delivery of health-care services.[36]

The TTH-MDS partnership was designed originally to set up a for-profit joint venture that would take over the hospital's laboratory operations and replace approximately 70 lab jobs with MDS's robotic AutoLab equipment. Joint ventures with the hospital sector, said MDS, would give it access to a "continuing stream of income, not just the one-shot equipment sales." Toronto Medical Laboratories (TML), the "Lab of the Future," went one step further, linking not only TTH, but five other hospitals to the enterprise, with the promise of more when the lab was fully functional. "Toronto Medical Laboratories is an excellent example of partnerships between hospitals and private industry," said Alan Hudson. MDS's laboratory information technology, a vital component of TML's automated approach, could integrate information systems in up to ten hospitals, while AutoLab would increase testing volumes by almost 290 percent. In all the excitement of TML's opening, no one questioned why the "continuing stream" of scarce public funds, once circulated within the hospital system, should be rerouted to enhance the revenue and profit margins of the joint venture.[37]

Osteopharm and the venture capital model

While the TTH partnership was an important one for MDS, it was the founding of a small company called Osteopharm, Ltd., that would more closely model the formal partnerships between MDS and a number of Canadian hospitals. Formed in 1993 as a joint venture between MDS, its venture capital arm MDS Health Ventures, and Toronto's Queen Elizabeth Hospital, Osteopharm was a biotechnology firm developing compounds for the treatment of osteoporosis. MDS and the hospital, an extended-care facility with a population of elderly patients, began preclinical testing of the compounds developed by Osteopharm in 1996. With an estimated 200 million people worldwide suffering from osteoporosis, and the market expected to reach $16 billion by the turn of the century, this investment by MDS positioned the company to realize significant future benefits. In addition, its partnership with an extended-care hospital provided a potential population base for clinical trials of Osteopharm's drugs.

In late 1996 Osteopharm was sold to Vancouver-based Biocoll Medical Corp. for $10 million in an unusual acquisition deal. Biocoll, a bone regeneration research and marketing company, was formed by Dr. James Trotman, a general practitioner, in 1980 and reformed during the early 1990s after merging with Stormin Resources, Inc. Biocoll's fortunes, which had faltered after clearance for its bone regeneration product was delayed by the U.S. Food and Drug Administration in 1993, were revived when the product received FDA approval two years later. With a laboratory in Seattle, Washington, Biocoll was stable but short of cash.

Discussions with MDS started early in 1996 when Biocoll went to the company hoping to raise between $5 million and $7 million. According to Louis Plourde, Biocoll's investor relations officer, MDS noted the "synergies" between the two companies and suggested Biocoll take over Osteopharm entirely. At this point Dr. Calvin Stiller, head of MDS's Canadian Medical Discoveries Fund, was brought on board to help engineer the deal.[38] Stiller, a professor of medicine at the University of Western Ontario and a well-respected physician in the scientific and medical communities, was appointed CEO of the new fund as well as CEO of the fund's manager, Canadian Medical Discovery Management Corp., an MDS subsidiary. Stiller also sat on a number of corporate boards, including Interhealth Canada, Oracle, Seragen Canada, and London and Midland Insurance. He was closely connected with MDS Inc., particularly its venture capital arms.

Stiller, who joined the Biocoll's board of directors as an officer, helped raise the company's profile among investors, as did the participation of MDS, which ended up with a 30 percent share of the company. Queen Elizabeth Hospital held 17 percent of shares, while the increasingly influential, government-backed − and MDS-managed − Canadian Medical Discoveries Fund (CMDF) held more than 10 percent. Thus, while Biocoll, about to be renamed GenSci Regeneration Sciences Inc., had managed a 100 percent takeover of Osteopharm, it was unclear who had taken whom.[39]

CMDF, which already owned 11.5 percent of Osteopharm, was set up in 1994 by six joint venture partners: MDS Health Ventures, the Professional Institute of the Public Service (PIPS), the federal government's Medical Research Council, Talvest Fund Management, Inc., and both CIBC Wood Gundy and CIBC Wood Gundy Capital. The fund was managed by the Medical Discovery Management Corp., another MDS arm, with a mandate to invest between $1 million and $3 million in health-industry companies in the early stages of research and product development. The Medical Research Council, which initiated the earliest discussions within the federal government leading to CMDF's creation, said the investment fund, with its focus on early stage product development, would "complement the existing MRC/PMAC Health Program." PMAC – the Pharmaceutical Manufacturers Association of Canada – represents U.S.-based drug companies, many of whom have developed clinical trial deals with MDS. By January 1996, with almost $200 million to invest, CMDF had come to the aid of eight companies, all of them subsidiaries of MDS Capital Corporation.[40]

Venture capital funding is a relatively new phenomenon in the Canadian health industry. Companies that started up in the health sector during the last twenty years confronted some daunting obstacles, including a lack of development capital in a notoriously high-cost industry. This was particularly true in sectors dependant on expensive technology and information systems. As MDS began to expand, it, too, was confronted by some daunting obstacles, including a market of limited size and scope, but one that held a great deal of promise as governments initiated massive cuts in health spending. What was needed was a concentrated effort and the harnessing of substantial capital to develop a private health industry where the business of buying and selling could unfold. Most venture capital funds involve a number of investors who pool their money, investing the capital in worthy start-up companies. The return to individual investors is in proportion to each one's stake in the pool. If the fund, which becomes an equity holder in the investee company, gets a return on the investment, it is divvied up among the fund's shareholders.

MDS Health Ventures was set up in 1988 specifically to address the problem of a small domestic market. The size of Canada's market did not limit the number of small entrepreneurs interested in developing a business, but it did explain the absence of investment capital. U.S. companies had overcome this obstacle long ago, and by the mid-1980s investment capital was the driving force in that country's health industry.

Ed Rygiel, a former engineer at IBM and chemical/medical giant W. R. Grace, and current president of MDS Capital Corp., senior vice president of MDS Corporate Development, and CEO of Drug Royalty Corp., another MDS/CMDF-funded offshoot, has been referred to as "the dean of health-care venture capital in Canada." According to Rygiel, in 1993 MDS Health Ventures was receiving funding proposals from 200 Canadian companies a year, plus another 150 from the United States. Rygiel's job was to filter through the proposed deals and pick the ones that held the most commercial potential. Not only did venture capital funding enable MDS to decide which companies did or did not attract development funds and allow it to expand its already sizable ownership share within the sector, but it also gave the company and its co-investors substantial control over decisions about the shape and character of the health sector as a whole. Venture capital funding, said Rygiel, "allows us to see what is happening in the marketplace much more broadly ... so we can take a look at the opportunities, the implications, and the best way to go forward." No longer was there a need to consult the Canadian people, a difficult and tedious process at the best of times. With a thriving, well-financed private sector, decisions could be more easily arrived at in corporate boardrooms.[41]

The factors which determine the company's venture capital investment decisions have less to do with the health-care needs identified by Canadians and more to do with the export potential of health-care products and services. As noted by Neville Nankivell of the *Financial Post*, "A health industries sector that builds on domestic success" is in a position to "penetrate export markets." If international markets wanted drugs and medical devices, expected to be worth almost $500 billion by the new century, then Canada's health-industry sector should begin producing drugs and medical devices. But if international markets started to favour health-information technology, Canadian companies, their investors, and political backers would have to reorient themselves – or be left behind in the global market. Thus in the late 1980s, health services led the investment "portfolios" of many such funds, a focus that shifted to the booming biotechnology market by early in the new decade.[42]

One of the attractions of CMDF was the status accorded the fund because of its "labour" sponsorship. Although PIPS was but one of the fund's six joint venture partners, its involvement was enough to trigger federal tax breaks for investors. Under federal rules, investors in labour-sponsored funds are eligible for a tax credit of up to 20 percent, plus matching credits in several provinces, for a maximum $2000 tax write-off on investments of $5000. It was a good deal for taxpayers who took advantage of the write-off, but it was an even better deal for MDS. The ability to direct public and private capital towards start-up companies, many (if not all) of which were already "investees" of one or more of the fund's corporate shareholders, presented a well of opportunities and minimum risk.

From 1988 to 1996 MDS had created, or helped create, no fewer than five venture capital funds across the country. In 1992 the company joined with Wood Gundy, Inc., Midland Walwyn Capital, and RBC Dominion Securities to form the Health Care and Biotechnology Venture Fund. Set up as a trust fund to generate capital gains and income for its unit holders, and thereby avoid paying taxes, the company was listed on the Toronto Stock Exchange, where it hoped to raise up to $50.4 million. Although MDS held only 10 percent of the venture fund, its promoter was MDS Health Ventures and its investment policies were developed jointly with MDS. In its first few months of operation, the fund invested $750,000 in MDS subsidiary Columbia Health Care, Inc., and $2 million in Hemosol, a Toronto-based biopharmaceutical company in which MDS had held a 22.7 percent equity stake since 1987. With a healthy injection of venture capital funds and the scandal surrounding HIV-tainted blood products, Hemosol, Inc., caught the attention of TSE investors after its blood substitution products entered clinical trials. In spring 1997, MDS was so enthused about the company's progress it increased its investment to 30 percent.[43]

In 1994 MDS established the Montreal-based Neuroscience Partners LP fund, the largest pool of health venture capital in Canada, with up to $105 million looking for private-sector investment opportunities. MDS's partners included the Royal Bank of Canada and the Caisse de depot et placement du Québec, as well as Manulife, Ontario Hydro Pension Fund, and the Manitoba Teachers' Retirement Fund. The biotech fund, which expected a rate of return of 25 percent over ten years, would invest in start-up, as well as established, companies inside Canada and internationally to support and market the work of a Montreal-based university research group that included scientists from across the country.

From the beginning MDS has relied heavily on public funds, money that has been drained from the publicly funded health sector across Canada. That money has fuelled the company's rapid growth and global expansion. It also has allowed MDS to fund other commercial health enterprises involved in biotechnology, pharmaceuticals and drug trials, home care, nuclear medicine, environmental health, and so on – and on. With more than $94 million directly invested by MDS Capital Corp. on behalf of the parent corporation, MDS is a major shareholder in more than forty health-care companies that together generate annual revenues in excess of $250 million. MDS's own annual revenues are predicted to reach well over $1 billion by the turn of the century. Another $400 million is managed by MDS, giving the company an enormous hold on significant aspects of the country's health sector. Its influence now stretches into every area of the health industry and is felt in every provincial capital in Canada, as well as in Ottawa. Its reach stretches not only across Canada, but throughout North America and around the world. MDS's strategy of sharing risks with the public while keeping the rewards in the pockets of its major investors has helped create one of the most powerful single players in Canada's health sector. For better or, more likely, for worse.[44]

FOURTEEN

Conclusion: Educating Canada

Cultural barriers, public education, and strategies to deregulate the activities of health corporations were among the subjects discussed at a March 1996 gathering in the small community of Montebello, Québec. Billed as the National Health Care Policy Summit, the meeting was sponsored by Liberty Health Canada, SHL Systemhouse Ltd. (a subsidiary of US-based MCI), MDS Inc., and the Canadian Medical Association. In attendance were Canada's elite business leaders, academics, and consultants, who convened in the stately Chateau Montebello for two days of discussion, problem solving, agenda setting, networking, and socializing.

The problems they discussed were government cuts in funding for health care (necessary, conference attendees agreed, to feed the debt/deficit) and Canada's subsequent inability to financially support the fundamental principles of national health-insurance embodied in the Canada Health Act. The solution the conference embraced was increased corporate involvement in Canada's health-care sector.

The conference sponsors were joined by an impressive array of corporate presidents and chief executives not normally associated with the health care industry, including those from BCE, Inc., Alcan Aluminum, Stelco, CP Rail, Trimac, and Nestle Canada. L. R. Wilson, chair and CEO of Bell Canada Enterprises (BCE), opened the summit by outlining the difficult task confronting the participants who, he said, represented a "wide range of views." This diversity was vital, Wilson emphasized, "because health care issues are too complex and interrelated for the public debate to be furthered by ideas coming from a single point of view." Their task, he said, was nothing less than "to take stock of where we are and to begin a process that will influence the course of public policy" in Canada's health-care sector.

But the summit was of one view, of one class, and of one mind. Few of the participants disagreed with the position of the summit's promoters, that corporate profits from health care were legitimate and, indeed, necessary to encourage investment. And investment was needed to save Canada's most cherished social program. Of the approximately fifty men and ten women gathered in the Chateau Montebello, thirty-one were from North America's powerful corporate community and another sixteen were doctors. The rest of the participants were like-minded individuals employed in public, publicly funded, or nonprofit institutions. The Canadian International Development Agency sent a representative to advise the meeting on how to export Canadian goods and services and privatization expertise to developing countries.

It was not a lack of interest that kept away representatives of Canada's 750,000 health-care workers or the country's 1.5 million union members or women, poor people, farmers, aboriginals, ethnic and visible minorities, youth, or religious denominations. Canadians from every walk of life, every region, from every generation, race, and religion, were expressing a heightened interest in discussions about their health-care system as the media daily bombarded them with stories declaring medicare was no longer viable in the global economy. Many were able and willing to discuss the problems facing medicare, including the greatest challenge ever to confront Canada's nonprofit, universally accessible health care system: the drive by corporations and individuals who wanted to turn the system into a new source of profits and revenues.

Not surprisingly, this challenge was not discussed at the National

Health Care Policy Summit. Conference participants focussed on access, but not the kind distressed Canadians were concerned about. Rather, the summit examined strategies to leap cultural and other barriers confronting large health corporations seeking access to a potential market worth billions of dollars. One idea put forward by participants was the creation of what was referred to as "internal markets" or, more plainly, domestic health markets composed of public buyers and private sellers of big-ticket items such as diagnostic and food services, high technology equipment, or insurance services. Such markets would provide corporations with access to a deep pool of public money that now was used – wastefully and inefficiently, they felt – by hospitals and other institutions to protect and ensure universal access to health care. As the published report on the summit proceedings tactfully put it, the creation of internal markets in the health-care sector "would blend the concept of market-based competition with the framework of a publicly-financed system."

BCE President L. R. Wilson phrased this idea even more delicately. Two very different approaches to health care had been developed over the years, he said. The Canadian approach stressed "community service and volunteerism," while the other approach emphasized the "enterprise system." He hoped that the conference would "discuss how key elements of these two very different approaches might best be brought to bear in designing the future of health care in Canada."

As the conference soberly noted, several steps had to be taken before such an merger could be achieved. First and foremost, Canadians had to face the fact that they could no longer support nonprofit, publicly funded health care. In his presentation to the summit, Frank Graves, president of Ottawa-based Ekos Research Associates, outlined the findings of a poll conducted by his company in preparation for the summit. The poll highlighted a key problem confronting the corporate community: public opinion. Sixty-one percent of Canadians surveyed in March 1996, Graves said, gave the health care system their stamp of approval, compared with only 19 percent who approved of the way the unemployment insurance system was run and 18 percent who approved of the way governments created (or didn't create) jobs. Undoubtedly it was another blow to conference attendees when they learned that only 6 percent of those polled said they preferred that private business be given responsibility for health care, compared to nearly 80 percent who said they wanted the federal government to either maintain or increase its role in the health-care sector. Fully 89 percent said Ottawa and the provinces should work together to improve the health-care system.

"This positive rating is a two-edged sword," Graves warned. "It is encouraging to think that we have a success story in such a crucial area as health care. At the same time, it is disconcerting to think that we are going to have to tell the public that this singular success story is no longer going to be available to them."[1]

Attitudes among Canadians have been identified by the corporate sector as a major hurdle that must be jumped if the profit potential of the health-care system is ever to be realized. Ideally, corporations would like public opinion lined up on their side, but if Canadians cling stubbornly to their romantic notions about sacred trusts and cherished social programs, the billions of dollars circulating in the health-care system will have to be siphoned out to the private sector through the back door. That back door is being opened by doctors, hospital administrators, and other champions of market medicine who are rerouting public dollars to the corporate sector, the new partners in the delivery of health care.

The Montebello summit renewed the foundations of an alliance among private insurers, employers, drug companies, consultants, entrepreneurial doctors, and a mix of information, biotechnology, medical, and industrial corporate giants. They sketched a blueprint for a health-care system that embraces profit and market competition beginning with public-private partnerships and the privatization of so-called noncore hospital services and services with a "low clinical content." These first steps must be taken, they felt, so that "public expectations about the health care system could be 'politely' managed" and people could get used to the idea of corporate, for-profit medicine.

What do Canadians want?

But is this the direction Canadians want to go? And if they don't want to travel this road, why aren't they rising up to protect the system they claim to cherish in poll after poll?

Previous generations in Canada rallied around a vision of health care that made sense to them and that clearly would benefit all equally. Many Canadians, despite lingering doubts, seem resigned to the proposals offered by corporations and by politicians who vow to "save" medicare by opening up the health sector to domestic and foreign investors. Proposals to maintain the system as it is are rejected – and for good reason. The system as it exists in the 1990s needs an overhaul. Often it seems as though Canadians know what kind of health-care system they want, but they are worried about whether the directions proposed by corporate Canada will get us there. But as Malcolm X once said, "If you don't believe you're on the right road, how do you think you'll get to the right place?" It is a question worth pondering.

Perhaps Canadians should begin with the picture of health care they would like to see established and work backwards from there. This is the way the corporate sector has achieved its goals. MDS, for example, decided at the beginning of the 1990s that it wanted revenues to reach $1 billion a year by the end of the decade. Every decision made by the company was reached with that objective in mind, and the goal has been achieved ahead of schedule. Canadians can learn a few things from corporations to help them reach their own goals in health care.

It's not hard to figure out what kind of system Canadians want. Support for the five principles of the Canada Health Act remains very high, with a general belief that public payment for insured services implies – or should imply – both public ownership and control of those services. Canadians want committed leadership and financial support from the federal government for health care. In the survey by Ekos Research, 84 percent of those polled rated equal access to health care for all Canadians and the quality of health-care services as the most important aspects of the system, while 60 percent rejected "queue jumping" by individuals able to pay for services.

Access, high-quality services, federal financial support and leadership, equity. That is what Canadians have said they want – there is no room for confusion on that score. The question, then, is how to get there.

Access and equity

If Canadians believe the private sector can protect access to health care, they should initiate a discussion with any American, insured or uninsured. The state of health care in the United States is dismal, with every effort to enhance access for the uninsured and under-insured a resounding failure. The number of uninsured Americans has increased each year since 1987, and the advent of managed care has only made matters worse. As corporations have increased their involvement in Canada's health-care system, access has decreased here, too. The corporate sector has successfully applied pressure on all levels of government to limit, not enhance, access to health services by Canadians. The delisting of services from public health plans, coupled with a refusal by provinces to cover new procedures and drugs, reflects the demands of the insurance industry, not of the Canadian people. Consequently, annual private-sector per capita expenditures have increased from $441 in 1987 to nearly $800 in 1997. These are figures that punish those who are the most vulnerable – people with chronic conditions, elderly people, aboriginal people, children, and employees who are not covered by supplementary benefits.

Yet insurance companies – who have demanded federal definitions of what is "medically necessary" to determine what will and won't be covered on public plans – are viscerally opposed to any regulation that would define what kinds of services they must provide and to whom. Proposals before the U.S. Congress, moaned Richard Huber, chair and CEO of Aetna Inc., would "establish a strict national policy for how all health plans must operate and what coverage they must provide." Huber, horrified at such a prospect, nonetheless heads a company that is expanding its presence in Canada's health sector and that is an active member of an industry calling for just such policies for public health insurance.[2]

Access and equity are important principles embraced by Canadians. But the road to achieving these laudable goals is in the public, not the private, sector. That doesn't mean maintaining the status quo – far from it. Equity does not currently exist in our health-care system, as the drastic cutbacks to aboriginal programs clearly demonstrate. Access is being eroded for all Canadians. But the politicians who are doing the cutting and expanding the role of the corporate sector continue to be reelected by voters who want access and equity to increase.

Canadians are quite capable of making the right decisions about health care, but only if they have information about how the system is working and only if that system operates in a transparent manner. Public disclosure of the activities of both the corporate sector and hospitals would benefit Canadians, allowing them to judge and evaluate the relationships that are emerging between public and private entities. The issue of transparency is fundamental to the ability of Canadians to make educated decisions about their health-care system.

The role of government

The course chosen by the federal government in the last ten years has led in a direction Canadians clearly reject. For all intents and purposes, Ottawa has shut down the federal health ministry and assigned the lead in most matters involving health care to Industry Canada. This ministry is headed by John Manley, a man well known to the chief executives in the corporate sector. While the names of health ministers are usually familiar to most Canadians, the men at the helm of Industry Canada are individuals with a low public profile. This is undoubtedly intentional. If Canadians knew of the damage inflicted on health care by Industry Canada, the minister's head would be on the chopping block.

Industry Canada is involved in ongoing and thorough discussions with corporate Canada about health care. In 1998 a ministry paper said the job of the federal government was to develop regulatory mechanisms that protect the health of Canadians without setting up barriers to the corporate sector. "The health of Canadians" is now defined in free trade agreements that have been signed and promoted by the federal government. The North American Free Trade Agreement and agreements under the World Trade Organization, said the paper's authors, had reduced tariffs "to the point where they are no longer a major issue." This is one of the most important factors in the increased activities of U.S.-based corporations in Canada. But many nontariff barriers remain, the paper said. These barriers are "patent policy, regulatory review processes and, increasingly, the use of 'managed care' instruments such as formularies, procurement and utilization policies by health care managers in government and the private sector."

According to Industry Canada, Ottawa must provide even longer patent periods for name-brand drugs and must remove even more regulations from the health industry. The managed care "instruments" referred to are the public tools that have allowed Canadians to exercise control over health care, tools that may be subject to future challenges by the corporate sector under the rules of free trade.

Federal and provincial governments claim that their hands are tied by the realities of globalization. The world economy, politicians plead, is forcing them to decrease their involvement in the domestic economy. But as Linda McQuaig and others have noted, the idea of the impotent state is a myth. In fact, governments are now more active in areas like health care and public policy than they have been in recent memory. They are actively dismantling the framework that allowed the state to act as a supplier of public services to Canadians and are working overtime to support global corporations eager to take over that function.

The policies of the federal government, and of most provincial governments, as well, are boosting the private-sector role in insuring and providing health services across Canada. At the same time, both federal and provincial governments are decreasing their regulatory and financial involvement. Concern about the future of Canada's publicly supported health-care system is rising for three main reasons:

● *Cuts to federal government financing.*
   Since 1986, cuts to federal transfers to the provinces for health have reached a cumulative total of almost $36 billion. Canada is racing to the bottom among twenty-eight OECD member countries in public spending on health care; it is fourth in overall public and

private spending. Over the last twenty years, private spending has risen from 23.6 percent of total spending to over 32 percent, while the public share has fallen to less than 68 percent. Private spending on health care now exceeds total federal government spending. Only 15 percent of public dollars spent on health come from the federal government, compared to 42 percent in the mid-1970s. The public-private split is expected to reach 60-40 by 1999.

As federal support for health continues to erode and as cutbacks in social-program funding increase, the factors that undermine good health – including increased poverty, unemployment, homelessness, hunger, and family breakdown – are being exacerbated. Provinces have responded to the withdrawal of federal support for health by delisting services and drugs from health plans or by refusing to insure new therapies and services that enable individuals greater autonomy, control over their treatments, and better health. Individuals face costs in the thousands of dollars to access these services, drugs, or medical devices. As Canada's population grows and ages, the need for services that are not now insured, from home care to nursing care, will continue to rise, further increasing financial barriers to medically appropriate health care.

● *Privatization.*

As provincial governments continue to cut health spending, there is a shift away from publicly funded and nonprofit care to for-profit payment and provision. Government spending cuts create a negative ripple effect throughout the economy. As fewer services are listed on public health plans, costs are shifted to employer-sponsored plans where premiums have been rising by 18 percent to 20 percent per year; individuals and families, particularly those employed by small and medium-sized businesses, are being forced to shoulder more and more of the cost for medical care. In addition, public funding cuts are leading hospitals to narrow the scope of their "core business." Outpatient services are being privatized and hospitals are contracting the corporate sector to provide a broad range of "noncore" services, including diagnostic and nutritional services and medical records management. To generate needed revenue, many hospitals are forming partnerships with large corporations to establish profit-making health companies.

● *Growing inequality.*

Privatization of both the payment and provision of health services is creating or supporting existing inequities across the country and between communities. A growing number of health-care services and products may become inaccessible to all except those who either have enough money to pay or are desperate enough to go into debt to get the care they need. Reaffirmation of a legislative and clearly defined federal responsibility for health care, along with increased federal-provincial cooperation, are urgently needed. Federal funding must be seen first and foremost as an enabler – in the same way that federal participation in infrastructure programs, for example, enables provinces to build wharves or highways – while reinforcing the ability of the federal government to maintain national standards.

What's the right road?

If in the 1960s Canadians could design a universally accessible and tax-supported health system composed of public payers and private providers, surely we can now create a better, more integrated system in the public sector, as well. Such a system could be based on federal criteria, with community input and control, providing a broad spectrum of primary health, social, and related services available in one location in each community. Community-based clinics could feature teams to deliver a full spectrum of care, from family counselling and physiotherapy to inoculations and eye examinations; an emphasis on prevention, health promotion, education services, and community development; and salaried remuneration of physicians and other health-care professionals.

But the framework for publicly insured health care in the Canada Health Act is outdated and inadequate. Funding health care through an insurance mechanism is failing to protect and maintain Canada's nonprofit system of delivery. It also undermines the creation of more affordable noninstitutional alternatives like community clinics and health-support services for in-home patients.

Studies indicate that tax-based health systems typically absorb two to three percentage points less of Gross Domestic Product (GDP) than social insurance models and tend to be more fully integrated at the community level. Canada, which has a tax-based system, is the exception to this rule: the use of insurance funding mechanisms and fee-for-service payments to physicians prevents us from maximizing the cost savings and efficiencies that characterize other tax-based models.

Insurance funding also undermines the development of an integrated community health centre model for basic health care. The term "integrated health-care delivery" has been seized upon by the U.S. corporate sector to describe a merger of payers and providers, whether those payers are workers' compensation or health insurers, and whether those providers are pharmaceutical or rehabilitation companies. In this scenario, health-care integration is facilitated by the manipulation of information systems tracking patients' use of prescribed drugs, medical products, and services – an information highway leading to restrictions on patient choices, the loss of autonomy and privacy, and the emergence of corporate-managed care.

The kind of health-care system Canadians want will not materialize unless and until we bring services, as well as payment, into the public sector. The insured system of financing health care is not affordable because for-profit companies are able to tap into the public pool on an equal footing with nonprofit providers. The pattern emerging in North America is an integration of not-for-profit and for-profit entities. The growing dominance of health corporations does not lead to better or more affordable health care. Nor does it eliminate the need for public funds, which are increasingly diverted to support the activities of the corporate sector. Another pattern that is emerging on the continent is the growing incidence of health-care fraud, which in the U.S. costs taxpayers an estimated $100 billion annually.

National drug strategy

While we are spending less on publicly supported hospital care, we are spending more on drugs. In 1975, 45 percent of all health dollars went to hospitals. By 1994 this had fallen to about 37 percent. In that same period, the cost of pharmaceuticals rose from 8.8 percent of expenditures to 15 percent – and most spending on drugs is out-of-pocket consumer spending. Drug costs have been growing at an average rate of 4.5 percent per year (a pace pharmaceutical firms complain is not quick enough).

For these reasons, in addition to a public-sector strategy for health care, Canadians need a National Drug Program reinforced by other measures to prevent inequities in drug coverage between provinces. The lack of a national strategy for new and existing drugs, along with the restrictive trade practices inherent in drug patent legislation such as Bill C-91, have led to increases in drug costs.

Access to drugs and drug-delivery mechanisms could be established as a right under the Canada Health Act, providing standardized drug coverage to all Canadians while also addressing the underlying supply-side factors (such as excessive pharmaceutical profits) that produce escalating drug costs.

To implement a successful and affordable National Drug Plan, developed in consultation with provincial governments, the following steps must be taken:

● *The repeal of Bill C-91 and a review of Canada's drug patent policies.* Rising drug costs are a consequence, in large part, of restrictive trade practices protecting patented drugs from fair competition from generic and alternative manufacturers. This protection places an extreme financial burden on individual consumers, hospitals, governments, and small employers, among others. Reinstitution of compulsory licensing potentially will save $4 billion over ten years. Generic brand preference legislation also may provide longer-term benefits to Canadians.

- *The centralization of drug purchasing in one agency for federal and provincial governments.* Bulk purchasing is widely used by U.S. insurers and employers as a practical method to lower prescription drug costs. Its use is long overdue in Canada. A central purchasing agency could be empowered to establish a lower "market value" on drugs, which would contribute to a reduction in drug prices, and to introduce a tendering process on bulk purchases. Limits could also be placed on pharmaceutical advertising, sales promotion, and similar activities.

Regulation of the drug industry needs to be increased, not relaxed. Drug companies may not be unethical, but it is safe to say they are not primarily guided by ethics. The testing of drugs on vulnerable patients, for example, is an ethical question that should only be raised within a very strict and regulated environment. It would benefit Canadians, as well, if caps were placed on the amount of money drug companies could extract from Canada's health sector.

What role for the corporate sector?

Corporations may not be able to establish and run the kind of health-care system Canadians say they want, but that does not mean they have no role to play whatsoever.

First and foremost, corporations should have an increased role in funding public health care through a more equitable tax system. Corporate taxes are diminishing in Canada, and this increases the burden on individuals to support public programs, including health. Yet the corporate sector is one of the main beneficiaries of publicly funded health. The benefits it receives include a healthier and more productive workforce and lower costs for businesses that provide supplementary health and dental plans. These are not insubstantial savings for companies doing business in Canada. If corporate taxes continue to decline – and, in fact, if they are not increased – the vision Canadians have for their health-care system will never materialize.

Because corporations are formed to earn profits, their role in the provision of services should come to an end. Canadians cannot afford to support both high-quality, accessible health care and profits at the same time. This is the crux of the matter confronting the nation as we head into the new century. It is the battleground of the near future, and Canadians will have to abandon their ambiguity about the issue if they want to realize the goals they have embraced for generations.

Solutions

It often appears there are no solutions to the problems that Canadians confront in the health-care sector. It often appears we are too far down the road to corporate control to turn back now. Things are too entrenched, the job is too mammoth. The kind of system Canadians want is too utopian in a world of globalized power.

It is useful to turn arguments against public health care on their heads. The plea of governments that they have no control in the global economy, for example, belies the fact that governments are more active in health care now than they have been since the creation of medicare. After all, it takes a powerful and committed government to withdraw $36 billion from the country's most cherished social program and embark on a concerted privatization scheme behind the backs of the electorate.

There is no single road to the kind of health-care system Canadians want and need. There are many roads, some of which are shorter than others. We've travelled the present road for more than a decade, and it is clear we're headed in the wrong direction. Like any lost traveller, it's time to abandon this road and choose another route.

NOTES

INTRODUCTION

1. Figures are from the Canadian Institute for Health Information, available on the Internet at *www.cihi.ca* (1996 and 1997 figures are forecast).

2. Jim Klein and Martha Olson, *Taken For a Ride* (Ho-Ho-Kus, NJ: New Day Films, 1996), documentary film.

ONE: HISTORICAL ALLIANCES

Invaluable sources for the first three chapters were:

Malcolm G. Taylor's *Health Insurance and Canadian Public Policy: The Seven Decisions That Created the Canadian Health Insurance System* (Montreal: McGill-Queen's University Press, 1978);

C. David Naylor's *Private Practice, Public Payment, Canadian Medicine and the Politics of Health Insurance, 1911-1966* (Kingston: McGill-Queen's University Press, 1986); and

C. Howard Shillington's *The Road to Medical Care in Canada* (Toronto: Del Graphics Publishing Department, 1972).

In chapter one I also referred to:

"A Brief Analysis of the Tentative Plan Suggested by the Health Insurance Commission," *CMA Journal*, March 1937;

Canadian Bar Association, "What's Law Got to Do With It? Health Care Reform in Canada," a report of the Canadian Bar Association Task Force on Health Care, 1994;

Canada. Royal Commission on Health Services,"The Evolution of Health Insurance in Canada,"in *Report of the Royal Commission on Health Services* (Ottawa: 1964-65);

Richard B. Saltman, "System reform in integrated health systems," *Physician Executive*, vol. 21, June 1, 1995.

TWO: 'A BRITISH COLUMBIA AND SASKATCHEWAN FREAK'

1. Blue Cross was the product of an experiment in prepaid hospital care begun in Dallas, Texas, in 1929 by a group of teachers. Within a year the plan had enrolled almost 3 million people in fifty-three plans across the country. In 1933 it was endorsed by the American Hospital Association.

The statistics on the dismal state of the public's health are from the Advisory Committee on Health Insurance Report, cited in Taylor's *Health Insurance and Canadian Public Policy*. The letters between Ian Mackenzie and Mackenzie King are also included in Taylor, as is much background material relating to the events in Saskatchewan.

Dr. Jason A. Hannah's comments were included in a letter to C. Howard Shillington, quoted in Shillington's *The Road to Medical Care in Canada*.

Robin Badgley and Samuel Wolfe, *Doctors' Strike: Medical Care and Conflict in Saskatchewan* (New York: Atherton Press, 1967).

THREE: THE FIGHT FOR NATIONAL MEDICAL INSURANCE

1. Expenditures included in estimates were for hospital services, publicly financed in both Canada and Britain, as well as physician and dental services, and prescribed drugs.

Taylor's *Health Insurance and Canadian Public Policy* includes a full discussion of the politics surrounding the implementation of the Hall report.

Canada. Royal Commission on Health Services, *Report of the Royal Commission on Health Services* (Ottawa, 1964-65).

FOUR: MEDICARE: THIRTY YEARS DOWN THE ROAD

1. Shillington, *The Road to Medical Care in Canada*.

2. John E. F. Hastings and Eugene Vayda, "Health Services Organization and Delivery: Promise and Reality," in *Medicare at Maturity: Achievements, Lessons and Challenges*, edited by Robert G. Evans and Greg L. Stoddart (Banff, AB: Banff Centre for Continuing Education, 1986).

3. Pat Armstrong and Hugh Armstrong, *Wasting Away* (Toronto: Oxford University Press, 1996), p. 163.

4. Ralph W. Sutherland, MD, and M. Jane Fulton, PhD, *Health Care in Canada: A Description and Analysis of Canadian Health Services* (Ottawa: The Health Group, 1992).

5. *Canada Health Act* and an overview of the Act (Ottawa: Health Canada/Santé Canada, March 12, 1996).

6. Pran Manga, "Health Care in Canada: A Crisis of Affordability or Efficiency?" *Canadian Business Economics*, Summer 1994; Colleen Fuller "A Matter of Life and Death: NAFTA and Medicare," *Canadian Forum*, October 1993.

7. Canadian Medical Association, "Toward a New Consensus on Health Care Financing in Canada: The Report of the Working Group on Health System Financing

in Canada," July 1993, and the CMA's "The Future of Health and Health Care in Canada: Restoring Access to Quality Care" (a background paper prepared for the CMA's General Council), August 1996; "Rethinking health care in Canada," *Globe and Mail*, December 2, 1994.

8. "Looking at Canada's health care: It's 'poised to self-destruct'," *Globe and Mail*, September 3, 1993.

9. "Magna boss wants to run health care for firm's workers," *Toronto Star*, September 25, 1995.

FIVE: RECREATING HEALTH CARE

1. Jeffrey I. Bernstein and Randall R. Green, *The Insurance Industry in Canada* (Vancouver: The Fraser Institute, 1988).

2. James Fleming, *Merchants of Fear: An Investigation of Canada's Insurance Industry* (Markham, ON: Viking Press, 1986).

3. Canadian Institute for Health Information, "Facts and Figures," available on the Internet (*www.cihi.ca*).

4. Jean Chretien, prime minister of Canada, interviewed by Peter Gzowski on *Morningside*, CBC, March 1, 1995; Thomas Walkom, "Surgery on medicare only will increase health costs," *Toronto Star*, March 14, 1995; Bob Cox, "Medicare returning to roots? PM sketches back-to-basics vision," *Winnipeg Free Press*, March 2, 1995.

5. "The Czech Republic – up, up and away?" *OTC News and Market Report*, April 1, 1996.

6. "Health care firms pick up the slack. Budget cuts open doors for entrepreneurs," *Toronto Star*, March 4, 1995.

7. "Insurer, government link urged," *Globe and Mail*, June 2, 1993.

8. Canadian Life and Health Insurance Association, Inc., "World Class Competitors," a submission regarding the North American Free Trade Agreement, presented to the sub-committee on International Trade, Standing Committee on External Affairs and International Trade, February 1993; *National Underwriter Life and Health: Financial Services Edition*, February 26, 1996; "Canadians face tough choices," *Life Insurance International*, March 1994, quoting Irene Klatt, director of health benefits, CLHIA.

9. "Playing the Trade Card," *New York Times*, February 7, 1997; CLHIA, "World Class Competitors."

10. "Partners being sought by Ontario health-benefits giant," *Globe and Mail*, August 25, 1994.

11. "Liberty International Canada Holdings Ltd. – Announcement," *Financial Post*, March 12, 1994; "International Managed Health Care – Announcement," *Financial Post*, April 16, 1994.

12. Thomas Walkom, "Inquiry could answer concerns over Blue Cross sale," *Toronto Star*, January 10, 1995, and "Province could block sale of Blue Cross if it wanted," *Toronto Star*, January 19, 1995; see also Walkom's series of articles on this subject; "Ontario Blue Cross and Liberty announce alliance," *Canadian Insurance News*, December 22, 1994; "The right medicine? Turmoil aside, selling Blue Cross was a good idea, supporters say," *Toronto Star*, September 26, 1995.

13. "Ontario Blue Cross and Liberty announce alliance," *Canadian InsurancE-*

NEWS, December 22, 1994; "OBC-Liberty International deal to close at midnight tonight," *Canadian InsurancE-NEWS*, January 31, 1995.

14. "Ontario Blue Cross, Liberty International Canada in new alliance; capital expansion plan unveiled," *PR Newswire*, December 21, 1994; "Liberty Health cuts workforce by 103," *Canadian InsurancE-NEWS*, April 12, 1996; "Ontario Blue Cross sold," *Globe and Mail*, December 22, 1994.

15. Judy Darcy, president of CUPE, letter to the Honourable Diane Marleau, federal Minister of Health, December 23, 1994; Julie Davis, secretary-treasurer of OFL, letter to Ruth Grier, Ontario Minister of Health, January 9, 1995.

16. "Blue Cross sale means 2-tier care, critic says," *Toronto Star*, December 23, 1994; "Second opinion needed," *Ottawa Citizen*, January 13, 1995; Thomas Walkom, "Blue Cross issue smooths over rifts in labor movement," *Toronto Star*, January 26, 1995, and "Province could block sale of Blue Cross if it wanted," *Toronto Star*, January 19, 1995.

17. Thomas Walkom, "Blue Cross sale can – and should – be put on hold," *Toronto Star*, January 24, 1995.

18. D. A. Wilson, U.S. Consulate in Toronto, "Canada: Selling Supplementary Insurance to Canadians," *Market Reports*, November 14, 1991.

19. "Dragging Out HMO Payments," *New York Times*, April 17, 1997; George Anders, *Health Against Wealth* (Boston: Houghton Mifflin Company, 1996); "Aetna Health makes first acquisition," *Globe and Mail*, December 12, 1996; "The Hospital for Sick Children – Announcement," *Globe and Mail*, December 13, 1996.

20. "Great West Life Assurance Company Claims Paying Ability Reaffirmed at 'AAA'," *PR Newswire*, May 7, 1996; "Power Financial shows steady earnings growth," *Financial Post*, August 1, 1996; "One Health Plan of Colorado and The Guardian offer new health insurance plans to Coloradans," *Business Wire*, February 10, 1998.

21. "Tax risk in AIDS insurance scheme," *Financial Post*, April 25, 1996.

22. "Playing the Trade Card," *New York Times*, February 7, 1997.

SIX: HEALTH CARE SERVICES:
THE POLITICS OF PRIVATIZATION

1. National Sector Team: Health Industries, "Canadian International Business Strategies – '97-'98," a report for Industry Canada, March 20, 1997. Available at Industry Canada's website (*strategis.ic.gc.ca*).

2. Ibid.

3. Kathy Megyery and Frank Sader (both of Québec-based Groupe Secors), "Facilitating Foreign Participation in Privatization," Occasional Paper 8, Foreign Investment Advisory Service of the International Finance Corporation and the World Bank, 1996.

4. Ibid.

5. "Constraints to the Export of Canadian Health Care Services," Industry Canada website (*strategis.ic.gc.ca*), undated.

6. "Healthy and Wealthy, A Growth Prescription for Ontario's Health Industries," report of the Health Industries Advisory Committee to the Honourable Ruth Grier, Ontario Minister of Health, March 1994.

7. "Private health care finds its niche," *Financial Post*, January 8, 1994.

8. Ibid.

9. "US health care giant quietly builds Canadian presence," *Financial Post*, August 13, 1996.

10. "Private health care finds its niche," *Financial Post*, January 8, 1994; Columbia Rehabilitation Centre brochure for the Backs That Work Program, Kelowna, BC.

11. *Inter-Corporate Ownership, 1996* (Ottawa: Statistics Canada, 1996); *Directory of Directors* (Toronto: Financial Post Co., 1993); "Sun acquires Canadian outpatient rehab company," *Business Wire*, December 12, 1995.

12. "See Sun. See Horizon. Watch them grow. And grow," and "Andy Turner wants the government out of health care," *New Mexico Business Journal*, April 1996.

13. "Leader of the Pack: With its pending $1.6 billion purchase of Horizon/CMS, Richard Scrushy's HealthSouth leaves the nation's other rehab providers in the dust," *Modern Healthcare* special report, August 4, 1994.

14. "Sun Healthcare to acquire Mediplex," *New York Times*, January 5, 1994; "See Sun. See Horizon. Watch them grow. And grow," *New Mexico Business Journal*, April 1996.

15. "Sun Healthcare Group announces fourth-quarter earnings," *PR Newswire*, February 28, 1997; "Sun Healthcare Group announces first-quarter earnings," *PR Newswire*, May 1, 1997; "Sun Healthcare to acquire Mediplex," *New York Times*, January 5, 1994.

16. "Sun Healthcare Group to acquire interest in Australian company," Sun Healthcare Group news release, June 4, 1997.

17. "Sun acquires Canadian outpatient rehab company," *Business Wire*, December 12, 1995.

18. Sun Healthcare Group, Inc., SEC Filing, Form 8-K, October 29, 1996; "US health care giant quietly builds Canadian presence," *Financial Post*, August 13, 1996.

19. "US health care giant quietly builds Canadian presence," *Financial Post*, August 13, 1996.

20. "Andy Turner wants the government out of health care," *New Mexico Business Journal*, April 1996.

21. "Columbia Health Care Inc. Announces Management Reorganization and Consolidation, Thomas Saunders Named President," *Canada Newswire*, October 7, 1997.

22. Sunder Magun, "The Development of Strategic Alliances in Canadian Industries: A Micro Analysis," *Applied International Economics*, October 1996.

23. Maude Barlow and Bruce Campbell, *Take Back the Nation* (Toronto: Key Porter Books, 1991), pp. 84-87.

24. Ference Weicker, "Survey of Canadian Pharmaceutical Companies," a survey for Industry Canada, March 31, 1996.

25. Julian Birkenshaw, "Business Development Initiatives of Multinational Subsidiaries in Canada," a report prepared under contract to Industry Canada, May 1995.

26. David MacKinnon, CEO Ontario Hospital Association, "Public-Private Partnerships in Health Care," speech to conference on public-private partnerships. November 25-26, 1996.

27. "Manitoba to use health info network," *AP Worldstream*, February 22, 1996; "Chasing medical markets; health care product manufacturing in Manitoba," *Manitoba Business*, June 1996.

28. "National Healthcare Manufacturing – First Quarter Sales Figures," *Canadian Corporate News*, September 30, 1996. More information on NHMC is available at the

company's website (*www.nationalhealthcare.com*).

SEVEN: THE MARKET GETS ANOTHER LEG UP

1. David U. Himmelstein, MD, and Steffie Woolhandler, MD, MPH, *The National Health Program Book: A Source Guide for Advocates* (Monroe, ME: Common Courage Press, 1994).

2. "Who is still uninsured in Minnesota? Lessons from state reform efforts." *Journal of the American Medical Association*, October 8, 1997.

3. Edmund Faltermayer and Rosalind Klein Berlin, "How to Close the Health Care Gap," *Fortune Magazine*, May 21, 1990.

4. Ibid.

5. Ibid.

6. Charles Andrews, *Profit Fever: The Drive to Corporatize Health Care and How To Stop It* (Monroe, ME: Common Courage Press, 1995).

7. "Efforts to implement national health reform in the United States," *Physician Executive*, March 1992; Robert Sherrill, "Medicine and the Madness of the Market," *The Nation*, January 9/16, 1995.

8. Mitchell Langbert and Frederick Murphy, "Health reform and the legal-economic nexus," *Journal of Economic Issues*, June 1995.

9. George Anders, *Health Against Wealth* (Boston: Houghton Mifflin Company, 1996).

10. Dr. Louis Sullivan, secretary of Health and Human Services, and Carl Schramm, president of HIAA, interviewed separately on *MacNeil Lehrer Report*, PBS, November 5, 1991 (transcript #4197); "Bush unveils health care plan / Not sure how to pay for it," *USA Today*, February 7, 1992.

11. "Health Insurers Run Scared, Expect Reforms to Shake Up Industry," *Los Angeles Times*, June 7, 1992.

12. Faltermayer, "How to Close the Health Care Gap," *Fortune Magazine*; Robert Laszewski of Liberty Mutual, interviewed on *MacNeil Lehrer Report*, PBS, November 5, 1991 (transcript #4197).

13. Andrews, *Profit Fever*.

14. "Helping Health Insurers Say No," *New York Times*, March 20, 1995; Anders, *Health Against Wealth*, 1996.

15. Edie Rasell and Marsha Lillie-Blanton, "The Clinton Plan: Hazardous to Our Health?" *Z Magazine*, January 1994; Langbert, "Health reform and the legal-economic nexus," *Journal of Economic Issues*, June 1995.

16. Vicente Navarro, *Dangerous to Your Health: Capitalism in Health Care* (New York: Monthly Review Press, 1993); Himmelstein, *The National Health Program Book*.

17. Himmelstein, ibid.; Edmund Faltermayer, "Health Reform: Let's Do it Right," *Fortune Magazine*, October 18, 1993 (interviews with Alain Enthoven and Paul Ellwood).

18. Suneel Ratan, "Why CEOs Aren't Buying the Plan," *Fortune Magazine*, October 18, 1993.

19. Langbert, "Health reform and the legal-economic nexus," *Journal of Economic Issues*, June 1995; Faltermayer, "Health Reform," *Fortune Magazine*, October 18, 1993.

20. Andrews, *Profit Fever*.

21. Navarro, *Dangerous to Your Health*; "Why Canada's Health Care System is No Cure for America's Ills," Michael Walker Heritage Foundation Report, November 13, 1989.

22. Steffie Woolhandler and David Himmelstein, "Universal Care? Not From Clinton," *New York Times*, June 12, 1994.

23. Laura McClure, "Labor and Healthcare Reform," *Z Magazine*, January 1994.

24. "U.S. firms start health-care reform," *Globe and Mail*, August 29, 1994; McClure, "Labor and Healthcare Reform."

25. "HMO fees rise sharply in a decade: Some changes are more than triple what they used to be a study says," *Orlando (FL) Sentinel*, May 4, 1997.

26. "The deal," *Hospitals and Health Networks*, June 5, 1996.

27. "Harvey and Louise Were Right, Sort Of," *New York Times*, November 24, 1996; "Health coverage lacking among minority Americans," *National Underwriter*, April 3, 1995; "GAO finds more children lack health insurance," *National Underwriter*, July 15, 1996; Anders, *Health Against Wealth*.

28. "When things go wrong" and "How Good is Your Health Plan?" *Consumer Reports*, August 1996.

29. "Memo to Members: Take the money and run?" *Consumer Reports*, August 1996; "In Hospital Sales, an Overlooked Side Effect," *New York Times*, April 27, 1997.

30. Susan Glazer, "Managed Care," *CQ Researcher*, April 12, 1996.

31. "U.S. Limits HMOs in Linking Bonuses to Cost Controls," *New York Times*, December 25, 1996; "Congress Weighs More Regulation on Managed Care," *New York Times*, March 10, 1997.

32. "Doctors' hope for their ills: Unions," *USA Today*, April 15, 1997; "Podiatrists to Form Nationwide Union; A Reply to HMOs," *New York Times*, October 20, 1996.

33. "Helping Health Insurers Say No," *New York Times*, March 20, 1995; "Congress Weighs More Regulation on Managed Care," *New York Times*, March 10, 1997; Glazer, "Managed Care"; "While Congress Remains Silent, Health Care Transforms Itself," *New York Times*, December 18, 1994.

34. Oxford Analytica Ltd., "U.S. health-care costs declining," reprinted in *Globe and Mail*, August 5, 1996; Murray Weidenbaum, "A new look at health care reform," *Vital Speeches*, April 1, 1995 (transcript of speech delivered to the Annual Health Policy Conference of the Quincy Foundation for Medical Research, February 9, 1995).

35. "Liberty Mutual increases managed care premium credit to 10%," *PR Newswire*, January 9, 1996.

36. "Bond portfolios beefed up in 1994," *Best's Review: Life-Health Insurance Edition*, October 1995.

37. Anders, *Health Against Wealth*; Himmelstein, *The National Health Program Book*; "While Congress Remains Silent ..." *New York Times*, December 18, 1994.

38. Anders, *Health Against Wealth*; "Cut Urged in Medicare Money to HMOs." *New York Times*, March 29, 1997; "PacifiCare Has Its Eye on the Prize," Los Angeles Times, August 6, 1996; "Medicaid Report Sees Costs Mounting at a Slower Rate," New York Times, January 17, 1997; "PacifiCare to Buy California Rival, FHP, for $2.1 Billion," New York Times, August 6, 1995.

39. "While Congress Remains Silent ..." New York Times, December 18, 1994; "Wealth and Power in the U.S. Health Care Industry," a paper produced by the Institute

for Health and Socio-Economic Policy (Oakland, CA), February 1996.

40. "Firms brace for rising health costs," USA Today, *October 9, 1997.*

41. "Health Care Costs Edging Up and a Bigger Surge is Feared," New York Times, *January 21, 1997.*

EIGHT: HE WHO PAYS THE PIPER ...

1. John Southerst, "OK Hillary, It's Our Turn," *Canadian Business*, December 1993.

2. "Medical empire building," *Winnipeg Free Press*, January 31, 1996.

3. "Actuaries give Canada five years to fix health care," *Financial Post*, February 23, 1996; Jason Clemens and Cynthia Ramsey, "Health Care Isn't Free – Even in Canada," *Fraser Forum*, October 1996.

4. David Gratzer, "Competition the best way to increase health-care efficiency," *Financial Post*, March 19, 1998.

5. "Financing Health Care Markets," a paper from Industry Canada's Health Industries Branch, November 12, 1996, available on the Internet (*strategis.gc.ic.ca*). The paper also looked at the advantages to the domestic health industry of free trade in services with the United States.

6. Cynthia Ramsey and Michael Walker, "A Thriving Health Care Sector Could Contribute to a Healthy Economy," *Fraser Forum*, October 1996.

7. Marc Law and Fazil Mihlar, "A Case for Repealing the Canada Health Act," *Fraser Forum*, October 1996.

8. "Who is still uninsured in Minnesota? Lessons from state reform efforts," *Journal of the American Medical Association*, October 8, 1997; "Blues for single-payer," *The Humanist*, November 1, 1994.

9. Clemens, "Health Care Isn't Free – Even in Canada."

10. "Private health care in Canada: savior or siren?" *Public Health Reports*, July 17, 1997.

11. Shahid Alvi, "Health Costs and Private Sector Competitiveness," report of a roundtable on health costs and competitiveness for the Conference Board of Canada, convened on May 25, 1994.

12. Judith L. MacBride-King, "Managing Corporate Health Care Costs: Issues and Options," report of a roundtable meeting of human resource and pharmaceutical executives for the Conference Board of Canada, March 1995; "Straight Talk and High Stakes," *Health Economics*, vol. 3, no. 4.

13. MacBride-King, "Managing Corporate Health Care Costs"; Alvi, "Health Costs and Private Sector Competitiveness."

14. "Straight Talk and High Stakes," *Health Economics*.

15. MacBride-King, "Managing Corporate Health Care Costs."

16. "Health pushes up benefit costs," *Financial Post*, September 28, 1996.

17. Shari Caudron, "Expose unveils health-care cost delusions," *Personnel Journal*, October 1996.

18. Ibid.; "Out of Control, Into Decline: The Devastating 12-Year Impact of Health-care Costs on Worker Wages, Corporate Profits and Government Budgets," a study by the Service Employees International Union, October 1992.

19. MacBride-King, "Managing Corporate Health Care Costs"; "Flexible Benefits and 'Managed Health Care': An Attack on Employees' Benefits," CUPE Research,

March 1996.

20. "Security company poised to lock out guards working at federal offices," *Ottawa Citizen*, October 24, 1996.

21. "Evolving for the Future, Part 4: Shifting Responsibility," *Benefits Canada*, report of a roundtable sponsored by the Health Alliance, a division of Astra Pharma, undated.

22. Ibid.; Lori Bak, "Benefits Canada assembles eight industry experts to tackle the thorny issue of implementing managed care in Canada," Eighth Annual Roundtable, *Benefits Canada*, 1996. Issues of this magazine are available at the website (*www.benefitscanada.com*).

23. "Evolving for the Future," *Benefits Canada*.

24. "Social Security costs: employers need open talks with governments," *Canada Newswire*, December 1, 1992.

25. "Employers join health-care fray," *Financial Post*, April 8, 1994.

26. "Straight Talk and High Stakes," *Health Economics*.

27. "Executives on front line of health care decisions" and "Migraine pill turns into a drug-plan headache," *Globe and Mail*, Report on Health and Pharmaceuticals, October 29, 1996.

28. "Big employers urge cutbacks in health costs," *Toronto Star*, July 20, 1995.

29. "Cost-effective delivery of drug plans sought," *Financial Post*, September 26, 1996; "Now it's the benefit crunch," *PROFIT Magazine*, Spring 1993; "Big employers urge cutbacks in health costs," *Toronto Star*, July 20, 1995; "Canadian companies are embracing managed care," *Globe and Mail*, October 29, 1996.

30. "Large employers agree: Health reform must be comprehensive, and should preserve marketplace improvements," *CanadaNews Wire*, June 2, 1994.

31. Ibid.; Donald K. Jackson, president and CEO of Laidlaw Inc., "Address to Shareholders," December 9, 1992.

32. Sandra Dudley, presentation at "Thrive and Survive in the '90s and Beyond with Public-Private Partnerships in Healthcare," a Toronto conference sponsored by The Canadian Institute, February 10 and 11, 1997. Ms. Dudley's quotes are from my own notes.

33. "Report reveals high rate of infant mortality," *Edmonton Journal*, November 23, 1996; "Infant mortality rates disputed," *Edmonton Journal*, November 29, 1996; "Alberta infant mortality rate on rise," *Globe and Mail*, January 17, 1988.

NINE: MANAGING CARE

1. Lori Bak, "Benefits Canada assembles eight industry experts to tackle the thorny issue of implementing managed care in Canada," Eighth Annual Roundtable, *Benefits Canada*, 1996. Issues of this magazine are available at the website (*www.benefitscanada.com*).

2. Mark Guest and Ric Walter of Sobeco, Ernst and Young, "Conspicuous by its absence," a report on the Benefits Canada website (*www.benefitscanada.ca*), September 1996.

3. Ibid.

4. Terry Thomason and John F. Burton, Jr., "The Workers' Compensation System in Ontario and British Columbia," unpublished paper.

5. Kyle Stone, "The best doctors money can buy," *Saturday Night*, September 1996.

6. Ibid. The Exclusion Paragraph also exempts medical check-ups required by a life, auto, or disability insurer or by an employer.

7. Shari Caudron, "Exposé unveils health-care cost delusions."

8. Ibid.

9. Rona Maynard, "The Pain Threshold," *Canadian Business*, February 1993; Fay Hansen, "Who gets hurt, and how much does it cost?" *Compensation and Benefits Review*, May 1, 1997

10. Company profile of Liberty Mutual Group, 1996, from *Hoover's Company Profile Database*, available over the Internet by subscription (*www.hoovers.com*); "Big dividends expected from rehab investments, occupational rehabilitation centers," *Best's Review: Life-Health Insurance Edition*, September 1994.

11. "Big dividends expected," *Best's Review*.

12. "Liberty Mutual to open 10-12 outpatient centers," *Boston Business Journal*, January 13, 1995; "Atlantic Health Group acquires three physical therapy facilities in Philadelphia area," *PR Newswire*, July 9, 1996; "Atlantic Health Group acquires U.S. Regional Medical Management Inc.," *PR Newswire*, February 15, 1996; "NYLCare/Healthplus and Liberty Mutual form strategic alliance for new workers compensation managed care program," *PR Newswire*, January 19, 1996.

13. Liberty Canada's Corporate Overview, undated. There is also much information at the Liberty Canada website (*www.liberty-health.ca*); "Liberty Mutual announces 1994 financial results," *PR Newswire*, April 19, 1995; "Workers Compensation Report," *Canada Newswire*, June 7, 1995; "Ontario Blue Cross, Liberty International Canada in New Alliance; Capital expansion plan unveiled," *PR Newswire*, December 21, 1994; "Big dividends expected," *Best's Review*.

14. "Rehabilitation on a roll; New insurance rules and cuts in health care spawn growth in private clinics," *Toronto Star*, September 12, 1994.

15. "Liberty pulls rehab firm funding," *Canadian InsurancE-NEWS*, June 12, 1996; "9 clinics are placed in the care of a receiver," *Toronto Star*, June 11, 1996; "Columbia seals IMHC deal," *Canadian InsurancE-NEWS*, August 16, 1996.

16. "The Compensation and Rehabilitation of Injured Persons in Canada," outline for Liberty Canada's study on workers' compensation *Unfolding Change*, August 12, 1994.

17. "New Approaches to Workers' Safety and Compensation in Ontario," Liberty Canada's submission to the Honourable Cam Jackson, Ontario Minister without Portfolio Responsible for Workers' Compensation Reform, March 1996; "Ontario plans Workers Comp reforms," *Journal of Commerce*, July 8, 1996; Liberty Canada's Corporate Overview, undated.

18. *Unfolding Change: Workers' Compensation in Canada*, 5 volumes (Toronto: Liberty Canada, June 1995).

19. Ibid.

20. Ibid.; "New Approaches to Workers' Safety and Compensation in Ontario."

21. Government of Ontario, "New Directions for Workers' Compensation Reform: Executive Summary," report of the Honourable Cam Jackson, Minister Without Portfolio Responsible for Workers' Compensation Reform, July 1996; "Report a step closer to WCB Privatization: Griffin," *Canadian InsurancE-NEWS*, July 31, 1996; "Industry beaming over Tory victory," *Canadian InsurancE-NEWS*, June 9, 1995.

22. "WCB reform a health issue: Wilkerson," *Canadian InsurancE-NEWS*, July 5, 1996.

23. "A Plan For the Organization and Delivery of Complementary Health Services in Canada," Health Resources Group Inc., April 1997, This plan was revised in May 1997.

24. ""Retirement deal for ex-WCB chief criticized," *Edmonton Journal*, July 22, 1998.

25. "Services offered no conflict, says hospital firm," *Calgary Herald*, May 17, 1997.

26. "Opening doors: A tangled feud over health-care services," *Maclean's*, June 16, 1997.

27. "Services offered no conflict, says hospital firm," *Calgary Herald*, May 17, 1997.

28. "First private hospital opens doors," *Calgary Herald*, September 29, 1997.

29. "Private hospital denied inpatients," *Calgary Herald*, October 4, 1997.

30. "Private hospital gets approval from college of physicians," *Calgary Herald*, August 16, 1997.

31. "Private health care in Canada: savior or siren?" *Public Health Reports*, July 17, 1997.

32. "Private clinic loses bid for overnight care," *Edmonton Journal*, December 6, 1997; "No overnight stays at private hospital," *Edmonton Journal*, December 11, 1997.

TEN: DEALING DRUGS IN CANADA

1. "Drug law cost set in billions, Report disputes Ottawa estimate," *Globe and Mail*, 17 November 1992; "Ministers reject use of loopholes to cut drug patents," *Globe and Mail*, March 6, 1997.

2. Canadian Health Coalition, "Need not Greed: A Brief to the House of Commons Standing Committee on Industry Review of Bill C-91," March 4, 1997.

3. "Drugmakers are discovering the high cost of cutting costs," *Business Week*, October 17, 1994.

4. National Sector Team: Health Industries, "Canadian International Business Strategies – '97-'98," a report for Industry Canada, March 20, 1997.

5. "Robust and Ready To Brawl," *Business Week*, January 8, 1996.

6. "Pharmaceuticals: take two aspirin and call in the morning," *Business Week*, January 9, 1995; "Drugmakers are discovering the high cost of cutting costs," *Business Week*, October 17, 1994.

7. "Lilly pays $4-billion for health firm," *Globe and Mail*, Report on Business, July 12, 1994; "Eli Lilly purchase of Rx Plus sets dangerous precedent," *Canada Newswire*, May 11, 1995; "Lilly Cuts Distribution Unit's Book Value by $2.4 billion," *New York Times*, June 24, 1997.

8. "Drug prices set too high," *Ottawa Citizen*, March 22, 1997; "Drugs cost us millions more than necessary," *Toronto Star*, March 23, 1997; "Drug review board was incompetent, ex-member says," *Ottawa Citizen*, March 27, 1997.

9. Rick Drennan, "Eli Lilly's purchase of a drug adjudicator is a tough pill to swallow for some in the benefits business," *Benefits Canada*, December 1995.

10. Ibid.

11. Ibid.; "Lilly Canada Acquires RxPlus: First Step into Managed Care," *Canada Newswire*, May 11, 1995; "Eli Lilly purchase of RxPlus sets dangerous precedent," *Canada Newswire*, May 11, 1995.

12. Drennan, "Eli Lilly's purchase of a drug adjudicator ..."

13. "U.S. firm to help Manulife cut plan costs," *Toronto Star*, November 3, 1995.

14. Steven G. Morgan, "Issues for Canadian Pharmaceutical Policy" (thesis, University of British Columbia, June 1996, rev. February 1997); "Drug costs will hit $9B, study says," *Ottawa Citizen*, February 6, 1997; "A decade of achievement in discovery and growth" (PMAC advertisement), *Globe and Mail*, March 5, 1997.

15. "RxPlus sold," *Benefits Canada*, January 1998.

16. Dr. David Caspari, director of medical and scientific affairs, Searle Canada (a unit of Monsanto Canada), "Public/Private Partnerships in Healthcare," a presentation to a Toronto conference organized by The Canadian Institute, February 10 and 11, 1997.

17. "IT and medicine, the perfect prescription," *Computing Canada*, June 9, 1997; "The Arthritis Society, Canadian Rheumatology Association and Searle Canada introduce innovative health education website," *Canada Newswire*, November 14, 1996; Caspari, "Public/Private Partnerships in Healthcare."

18. Sandy Lutz, "Home-care companies' offerings take off," *Modern Healthcare*, June 3, 1991.

19. "The Numbering of America: Medical ID's and Privacy (Or What's Left of It)," *New York Times*, July 26, 1998.

20. "Amex to sell information about consumers," *USA Today*, May 19, 1998.

21. "The Numbering of America," *New York Times*.

22. Ralph Nader and Lori Wallach, "GATT; NAFTA, and the Subversion of the Democratic Process," in *The Case Against the Global Economy and for a Turn Toward the Local*, edited by Jerry Mander and Edward Goldsmith (San Francisco: Sierra Club Books, 1996) p. 99.

23. "CBS Online Health Sector Consultation: Health Industries, Canadian Biotechnology Strategy On-Line," Canadian Biotechnology Strategy Taskforce website (*strategis.ic.gc.ca*), April 14, 1998.

24. "Research without patient consent now allowed; Change applies only in life-threatening situations with pre-approved studies," *Minneapolis-St. Paul Star Tribune*, November 5, 1996.

25. "Experimental Drug Use Debated," Associated Press, *Newsday*, December 24, 1996.

26. Canadian Biotechnology Strategy Taskforce website.CBS Health Sector Consultation.

27. Ibid.

ELEVEN: TRAFFIC ON THE INFORMATION HIGHWAY

1. "Towards a Canadian Health Iway: Vision, Opportunities and Future," CANARIE, Inc., undated

2. "FoxMeyer and Evans Health Group launch FoxMeyer Canada Inc. to serve health care delivery system," *Canada Newswire*, June 28, 1994.

3. "FoxMeyer Canada nominates six Canadian and American business leaders to

Board of Directors," *Canada Newswire*, January 17, 1995.

4. "FoxMeyer Canada makes strategic investment in ABEL Computers," *Canada Newswire*, June 1, 1995; "FoxMeyer Canada signs contract with Ontario Public School Boards' Assn to manage pharmacy benefits," *Canada Newswire*, August 23, 1995; HealthStreams Technology, Inc., CanCorp Plus Database, April 21, 1997. CanCorp Plus Database is a filing company that accepts annual reports and other information from companies and makes them available for prospective investors to peruse.

5. CanCorp Plus Database, April 21, 1997; "FoxMeyer Canada Inc., signs agreement in principle to acquire 1st Group Inc.," *PR Newswire*, January 8, 1996.

6. CanCorp Plus Database, April 21, 1997; "FoxMeyer Canada forms electronic health care network," *The Wall Street Transcript*, August 21, 1995.

7. CanCorp Plus Database, April 21, 1997; "IT and medicine, the perfect prescription," *Computing Canada*, June 9, 1997.

8. "Is FoxMeyer Out-Foxing Wall Street?" *The Dorfman Report*, CNBC, November 20, 1995 (transcript); "FoxMeyer sued for US$198 million," *South China Morning Post*, November 28, 1996; "FoxMeyer Health Corp. sells its position in FoxMeyer Canada Inc.," *Business Wire*, September 10, 1996; "FoxMeyer Canada Inc.; Gordon Capital Corp.; Marleau Lemire Inc.; FoxMeyer Health Corp.," *Mergers and Acquisitions Canada*, November 1, 1996.

9. "HealthStreams hunts for complementary alliance," *Financial Post*, May 22, 1997.

10. "How smart is SmartHealth?" *Winnipeg Free Press*, March 9, 1995.

11. "Manitoba to use health info network," *Associated Press Worldstream*, February 22, 1996,; Director biographies, CANARIE, Inc., 1996.

12. "EDS Canada and SmartHealth team up to tackle global health information network market," *Presswire*, June 13, 1997.

13. "EDS acquires Value Health Management," EDS news release (online at *www.eds.com*), March 6, 1997.

14. "EDS signs contract with Texas to redesign eligibility processes in state's Health and Human Services and Workforce Programs," EDS news release, August 18, 1997.

TWELVE: OUTSOURCING THE HOSPITAL SECTOR

1. Figures from the Canadian Institute of Health Information (CIHI), available on the Internet (*www.cihi.ca*). 1996 and 1997 figures are forecast.

2. "Outsourcing Boom: Survey shows more hospitals turning to outside firms for a broad range of services," *Modern Healthcare*, September 1, 1997.

3. Tony Dagnone, presentation to "Thrive and Survive in the '90s and Beyond with Public-Private Partnerships in Healthcare," a Toronto conference sponsored by The Canadian Institute, February 10 and 11, 1997.

4. "Three hospitals to close, 2000 jobs in jeopardy," *London Free Press*, February 17, 1997.

5. Henry J. Pankratz, deputy chairman Ernst & Young, "Private sector involvement in Canadian health care," a presentation to "Thrive and Survive in the '90s"; John Stirling, Meighen Demers law firm, "How to structure a win/win public-private deal," a presentation to the same conference.

6. "One-stop shopping," *Modern Healthcare*, November 25, 1996.

7. For an excellent discussion of privatization, see Paul Starr, "The Limits of Privatization" (Washington, DC: Economic Policy Institute, 1987).

8. "Measuring Value in Healthcare: The Quality Factor," *Compensation and Benefits Review*, September 18, 1997; Tyler L. Chin, "Outsourcing," *Health Data Management*, August 19, 1997.

9. Jim Weil, "How do Canadian hospitals do it? A Comparison of Utilization and Costs in the United States and Canada," *Hospital Topics*, vol. 73, January 1, 1995.

10. Chin, "Outsourcing."

11. Company profile on HBOC web page (*www.hboc.com/about/profile.html*); *"Canadian healthcare executive to lead HBOC's oursourcing efforts in Canada,"* HBOC News, *June 3, 1997; "HBOC expands Canadian services to include outsourcing,"* HBOC *Industry News (on the Internet at* www.hboc.com/news/ indnews/ind208.htm*), April 25, 1996.*

12. *Starr, "The Limits of Privatization."*

13. *"In Hospital Sales, an Overlooked Side Effect,"* New York Times, *April 27, 1997.*

14. *"A Delicate Balancing Act,"* Modern Healthcare, *March 13, 1995; "In Separate Studies, Costs of Hospitals Are Debated,"* New York Times, *March 13, 1997.*

15. *"Who protects public as hospitals aim for profits?"* USA Today, *December 17, 1996; Robert Kuttner, "Columbia/HCA and the Resurgence of the For-Profit Hospital Business,"* New England Journal of Medicine, *August 1, 1996; "U.S. Expands Search of Columbia/HCA in Texas,"* New York Times, *March 21, 1997.*

16. *"Blue Cross merger would put competition in fast lane,"* Cleveland Plain Dealer, *March 16, 1996.*

17. *Ibid.; "Blue Cross warns Ohio plan not to sell to Columbia,"* New York Times, *June 14, 1996; "Blue Cross questions purchase of Ohio plan by Columbia/HCA,"* New York Times, *September 21, 1996; "Columbia sings the (Ohio) Blues,"* Hospitals and Health Networks, *April 5, 1997.*

18. *"California Challenges Deal on Nonprofit Hospital,"* New York Times, *November 9, 1996.*

19. *Kuttner, "Columbia/HCA and the Resurgence of the For-Profit Hospital Business."*

20. *Thomas Walkom, "Health care cuts spell p-r-o-f-i-t for doctors,"* Toronto Star, *March 25, 1995.*

21. *Tom Fennell, "The privates' progress: the role of business in health care is growing,"* Maclean's, *special report, December 2, 1996.*

22. *"First private hospital opens doors,"* Calgary Herald, *September 29, 1997; "Canada Notes: Health-care showdown,"* Maclean's, *May 26, 1997.*

THIRTEEN: MDS INC., CANADA'S HOMEGROWN BEHEMOTH

1. Information on MDS came from the company's website (*www.mdshealth.com/i_div.htm* and *www.mdsintl.com/mdshvcc*).

2. Company annual reports; "MDS plans venture to do lab work for hopsital; other deals expected due to health cuts," *Toronto Star*, March 28, 1995.

3. MDS Inc., CanCorp Plus Database, December 2, 1996; "MDS records highest revenues and earnings in its 27-year history," *Canada Newswire*, January 16, 1997.

4. Dr. Keith Walker, director of pathology, Greater Victoria Hospital Society, "Delivery of Laboratory Diagnostic Services: A Presentation on Behalf of the Public Hospital," August 1995

5. *Financial Post* Corporate Survey: MDS, 1996; "Much to be Proud of in 1993 Annual Report," special 1993 annual report edition of *Perspective* (published by MDS Health Group Ltd.), March 1994; "Building a Company: A Capsule History," *Perspective*, May 1994; "From Labs in Ontario to International Diversification," *Perspective*, February 1994.

6. "Laboratory Services Review: Final Report," Ontario Ministry of Health, February 1994; "Review of Diagnostic Services: A Report to the Minister of Health of the Province of British Columbia," September 1993 (the Kilshaw Report).

7. "More tests than ever flow to Ontario labs," *Globe and Mail*, December 26, 1991.

8. Ibid.; "MDS will make a healthy recovery," *Financial Times*, August 2, 1993.

9. "Laboratory Services Review: Final Report," Ontario Ministry of Health, February 1994; the Kilshaw Report.

10. "Building the Future Together," *Perspective*, 1994; "MDS Laboratories," *Perspective*, May 1994; "Lab company sees opportunity in austerity," *Financial Post*, July 30, 1994.

11. "MDS Laboratories: 25 Years of Service and Accelerating Chanage," *Perspective*, May 1994.

12. "Profit down, MDS may cut 200 jobs," *Toronto Star*, January 26, 1994; "Top 5 officers at MDS take cut in income," *Toronto Star*, March 24, 1994; "MDS sees sharp gain in revenue," *Toronto Star*, September 23, 1993.

13. "Medicare? Gotta Love It," *Canadian Business*, June 1997; "Lab company sees opportunity in austerity," *Financial Post*, July 30, 1994.

14. "Soaring health costs spur MDS expansion; anticipating cuts led to automated lab," *Toronto Star*, April 27, 1994.

15. "MDS AutoLab: First U.S. Installation," *Canada Newswire*, November 7, 1996; "Automated Tooling Systems, Inc." *Investor's Daily*, March 21, 1997.

16. "Innovation daughter of necessity at lab firm," *Toronto Star*, July 13, 1993.

17. Information on MDS locations from the company website (*www. mdsintl.com*).

18. *Perspective*, special 1996 annual report edition, February 1997.

19. Louise Kinross, "Forging Alliances: Partnerships Between Hospitals and the Private Sector," *Canadian Health Care Management*, February 1993.

20. "Doing More With Less: A Leadership Opportunity," *Perspective*, June 1993; "Don't shut down private labs," *Financial Post*, May 26, 1993; Thomas Walkom, "A 'common sense' dilemma on medical lab testing," *Toronto Star*, November 14, 1995.

21. "Doing More With Less," *Perspective*.

22. "Western Labs Key to Health Group Network," *Perspective*, September 1994.

23. Kilshaw Report.

24. Kilshaw Report.

25. "$20m boost for technology," *Vancouver Province*, September 16, 1994; the Honourable Glen Clark, B.C. minister of Employment and Investment, speech at the MDS launch, September 15, 1994.

26. "Sharing the Burden: Health Care and the Private Sector," *Perspective*, Spring 1987.

27. Robert L. Michel, MDS-Hudson Valley Laboratories, Inc., "A For-Profit Joint

Venture Involving Hospitals and a Commercial Laboratory," undated article.

28. "Corning Lab Services to Acquire U.S. Clinical-Laboratory Business of MDS," *PR Newswire*, January 13, 1992; "Corning Will Plead Guilty to Medicare Fraud," *New York Times*, October 10, 1996; "MDS U.S. Hospitals Partnership Grows Again," *Canada Newswire*, February 5, 1997; Michel, "A For-Profit Joint Venture ..."

29. "1199 Calls on Vassar Brother's CEO Mullahey to Explain the Exclusive Relationship Between For-Profit MDS with Not-for-Profit VB Hospital," *PR Newswire*, July 16, 1997.

30. Canadian Institute for Health Information, "Facts and Figures," on the Internet (*www.cihi.ca*), including data on "Public Sector Health Expenditures by Province/Territory, Canada 1975-1997," and "Private Sector Health Expenditures by Province/Territory, Canada 1975-1997."

31. James H. Stonehouse, Alan R. Hudson, and Michael J. O'Keefe, "Private-Public Partnerships: The Toronto Hospital Experience," in *Strategic Alliances in Health Care: A Casebook in Management Innovation*, edited by Peggy Leatt, Louise Lemieux, Charles and Catherine Aird (Ottawa: Canadian College of Health Care Administration, 1996).

32. "Hospital embraces computers in quest to improve 'product'," *Financial Post*, October 15, 1994.

33. Stonehouse, "Private-Public Partnerships."

34. Ibid.

35. "London hospital forms partnership in private sector to help control health care costs," *Canada Newswire*, February 3, 1994.

36. Stonehouse, "Private-Public Partnerships"; "$2 Million Searle Chair in Cardiovascular Research Established at The Toronto Hospital," *Canada Newswire*, February 12, 1997. Searle contributed nearly $4 million to fund medical research and education at the University of Toronto, money that directly benefitted TTH as the university's teaching hospital. What Searle would receive in return was not mentioned.

37. "The Toronto Hospital and MDS Inc. Unveil Lab of the Future," *Canada Newswire*, April 16, 1997.

38. "Biocoll acquires all outstanding shares of Osteopharm," *BioTech Financial Reports*, February 1997,; "Osteopharm; Biocoll Medical Corp.," *Mergers and Acquisitions Canada*, January 1, 1997; "FDA ruling gives some bite to Biocoll," *Financial Post*, November 26, 1996; "We're Back," *Interhealth News and Views*, August 7, 1996.

39. "FDA ruling gives some bite to Biocoll," *Financial Post*, November 26, 1996; Biocoll Medical Corp., CanCorp Plus Database, August 1, 1997.

40. Canadian Medical Discoveries Fund, Inc., prospectus, December 7, 1994; "Medical Research Council to identify best projects for new medical discoveries fund," *MRC Communique*, December 15, 1994.

41. "Canada: Visionary with Clout – Ed Rygiel, MDS Health Group, Ltd.," *Financial Post*, September 17, 1996; "The Start-up Star Who Bats .900," *Canadian Business*, March 1993.

42. Neville Nankivell, "How to improve the marketing of medical technologies," *Financial Post*, May 10, 1994; "Health Sciences offer strong earnings potential," *Financial Post*, February 15, 1996.

43. "Biotech fund with a twist," *Financial Post*, January 31, 1992; Health Care and Biotechnology Venture Fund, CanCorp Plus Database, June 26, 1997; "High-soaring

biotech funds take 16% nosedive," *Financial Post*, August 18, 1992; "MDS increases investment in Hemosol," *Canada Newswire*, April 10, 1997.

44. "Health sciences offer strong earnings potential," *Financial Post*, February 15, 1996; information on MDS Capital Corp. is from the company's website (*www.mdsintl.com/mdshvcc*).

FOURTEEN: EDUCATING CANADA

1. "Making a Good Health Care System Better: Public-Private Partnering," proceedings of a National Health Care Policy Summit, March 18-19, 1996.

2. Richard L. Huber, "Viewpoint: In Health Insurance, Shades of 1994," *New York Times*, August 9, 1998.

INDEX

development of, 219-20; founding of, 216; and health information applications, 211; and MDS Inc., 248. *See also* FoxMeyer

Hemosol, 272

Heward, Bob, 94

Hewlett-Packard, 112, 137

Hill, Grant, 83

Hillhaven Corporation, 104

HMO Act (U.S.), 123, 132

HMOs. *See* health maintenance organizations

home infusion therapy, 202

Horizon Health Care Corporation, 104, 105

Hospital and Diagnostic Services (HIDS) Act, 39-40, 41

hospital insurance: in 1970s, 80; and competition, 31, 34, 35, 36; early types of, 18, 19; national (1955), 39-41; provincial, 33, 38, 39; and TCMP, 39. *See also* Blue Cross

Hospital Medical Records Institute, 112

hospitals: and bed closures, 146-47; and Blue Cross, 33-34; closures of, 8, 68, 75, 93, 101; core missions of, 229-30; and corporations, 147-49; and delisting of services, 228-29; and early health insurance, 17-18; for-profit, 185-86, 227; lack of, 13; and lengths of stay, 146-47; in Manitoba, 115-16; and medicare, 13, 15, 74; in Ontario, 88, 89; and partnerships, 239-45; private operation of, 244; private spending on, 285; and privatization, 228; and provincial funding, 112, 227; and provincial jurisdiction, 227-28; public and private, 226-27; in Québec, 68; and revenues, 266-67; and services, 227; status of, 239-40; union, 19. *See also* hospital insurance; outsourcing; names of hospitals

hospitals (U.S.): and Diagnostic Related Groupings, 125; and HMOs, 133, 146; takeovers of, 239-40

Hospitals of Australia Corp., 244

Hotel de Health (Edmonton), 244

Hôtel Dieu (Chatham, N.B.), 18

Huber, Richard, 279-80

Hudson Shared Services (HSS), 261-63

Hudson, Alan, 267, 268

IBM, 112, 271

Imasco, 205

Imperial Tobacco, 205

IMS: and Health-Streams, 211; and IBM, 211

income, Canadians', 31, 54-55

income, physicians': in 1920s, 20; in 1930s, 20, 21, 25; in 1940s, 33; in 1950s, 33; and CMA, 21; and insurance industry, 36; and insurance, 19, 22, 31-32, 33; and medicare, 72; in U.S., 72. *See also* individual provinces

Industry Canada: and domestic-foreign alliances, 100, 101, 186, 224-25; and health care, 280-81

infant mortality rates: in Canada, 27-28, 164; in U.S., 149-50

information highway: description of, 210-11; and patient information, 211-12

information technology and telecommunications (IT&T) industry: and health information industry, 212-13; market, 210. *See also* health IT&T industry; information highway

Inmark Group, 184

Institute for Clinical Evaluation, 221

Institute of Medicine, 239-40

Institute for Research on Public Policy (IRPP), 148-49

insurance: automobile, 88; consortiums, 39; enrollment, 34, 37, 48, 52, 53, 68, 69, 87, 88; general, 80; health (*see* health insurance; medicare); home, 80-81; indemnity, 36, 43; life, 31, 80-81; social, 14-15, 16, 24; syndicates, 39; and the uninsurable, 41, 50, 52; and the uninsured, 34, 48, 52, 88

Insurance Bureau of Canada (IBC), 171-72: in Ontario, 182